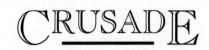

CRUSADE

CRUSADE

The Official History of the American Cancer Society®

WALTER S. ROSS

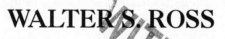

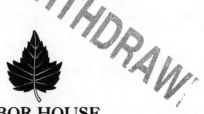

ARBOR HOUSE
NEW YORK

Manufactured in the United States of America

10 9 8 7 6 5 4 3 2 1

Library of Congress Cataloging in Publication Data

Ross, Walter Sanford, 1916–
    Crusade : the official history of the American
Cancer Society.

    1. American Cancer Society—History   2. Cancer—
Research—United States—History.   I. Title.
RC276.R67   1986   616.99'4'006073   86-28701

ISBN: 0-87795-811-4

The author gratefully acknowledges permission to quote from the following sources:

Quote from *Journal of the American Medical Association* by R. Doll, vol. 251, 1984. Copyright © 1984, American Medical Association. Reprinted by permission.

From *Reach to Recovery* by T. Laser and W. K. Clarke. Copyright © 1972 by Simon & Schuster. Reprinted by permission.

From "The Pap Smear," by D. E. Carmichael. Copyright © 1973. Reprinted by permission of Charles C. Thomas, Publisher, Springfield, Illinois.

Quote from *The New York Times*, "Cigarettes Found to Raise Death Rates in Men 50 to 70," by Lawrence E. Davies, of June 22, 1954. Copyright © 1954 by The New York Times Company. Reprinted by permission.

To the 2,500,000 volunteers of the American Cancer Society—more than two of every one hundred U.S. volunteers—in honor of the organization's seventy-fifth anniversary.

The purpose of this book is to illustrate how the American Cancer Society became the world's largest volunteer health organization. It tells why volunteers started the Society and how they made it grow. It is designed to provide a view of how volunteers go about setting the organization's goals and achieving them. It also offers insight into what the Society does and how it works; and why several of its major programs and policies gave rise to and/or settled some bitter professional and public controversies.

Americans of all ages, all conditions, and all dispositions, constantly form associations. . . . not only commercial and manufacturing companies in which all take part, but associations of a thousand other kinds . . . to give entertainments, to found establishments for education, to build inns, to construct churches, to diffuse books, to send missionaries to the antipodes; and in this manner they found hospitals, prisons, and schools. I have often admired the extreme skill with which the inhabitants of the United States succeed in proposing a common object to the exertions of a great many men, and in getting them voluntarily to pursue it.

Nothing . . . is more deserving of our attention than this sector. . . . The health of a democratic society may be measured by the quality of the functions performed by private citizens.

—Alexis de Tocqueville
Democracy in America

Contents

Preface   xiii
Acknowledgments   xix

PART ONE
Target: Cancer

I	Halfway to Victory	3
II	Cancer Risk	9
III	Organizing the Attack	15
IV	Moving Up	23
V	Pullback and Advance	28
VI	Transformation	33
VII	The New Executive Vice-President	41

PART TWO
Controversies

VIII	The Smoking Gun	47
IX	The Gun Goes Off	56
X	The Government Joins the Battle	64
XI	The Cell Yields a Secret	76
XII	The Selling of the Cell	84
XIII	Breast Cancer: Can Women Be Protected?	94
XIV	Breast X-Ray: Can It Save Lives?	101
XV	"Purposeless Mutilations"?	108
XVI	Developing a Clearer Picture	114

PART THREE
Cancer Research

XVII   Cancer Research: The Black Hole   121
XVIII   Research: The End of Cancer   125
XIX   Clinical Research: To Help the Cancer
            Patient   143
XX   ACS International   153

PART FOUR
Human Values

XXI   Reach to Recovery   161
XXII   The Warm Hand of Service to Patients:
            Volunteers Create Their Own Programs   172
XXIII   Life After Cancer   179
XXIV   Affirmative Action: Cancer in Minorities   183

PART FIVE
Public and Private Issues

XXV   Crusade   193
XXVI   United Way or a Better Way?   198
XXVII   ". . . Without Representation"   206
XXVIII Cancer Becomes a National Priority: The
            National Cancer Acts   210
XXIX   Public Issues   223
XXX   The Record   236

Appendix A   243
Appendix B   246
Appendix C   249

Appendix D	251
Notes and References	255
Index of Names	273
Index of Subjects	279

Preface

The powerful spirit of voluntarism that Tocqueville discerned in the United States in the 1830s has not only endured, but intensified. Nowhere else are peaceable voluntary associations so numerous, so widespread, or so varied as in the United States of America.

And nowhere else on earth do so many people get together on their own to help one another. Ninety-two million Americans volunteer to work for at least one organization.

The fact that voluntarism flourishes here more strongly than elsewhere reflects the conditions under which the country began: A handful of people with limited individual resources volunteered to come to this land and pit themselves against a hostile, often savage environment. They were forced to help each other in order to survive.

They banded together in self-defense. They worked shoulder to shoulder to help their neighbor build his barn. Then they organized themselves into a volunteer fire department to save it.

They shared their wealth with their churches through tithing. And many went far beyond this; before there were income taxes, American capitalists led the world in endowing libraries, educational foundations, universities, art museums, and symphony orchestras. In more recent times, U.S. income and property tax laws have been written to encourage public philanthropy by all Americans; few other countries give such favorable fiscal consideration to humanitarian impulses.

Thus, spontaneous social cooperation became woven into the fabric of the country. It is a responsible third sector of our society, neither private enterprise nor government, but equal to both and performing functions that they cannot.

Since volunteers create their own organizations, they set their own agendas. Perceiving needs, they attempt to fill them. They improve the quality of life.

Voluntarism is also an escape valve for society. It vents pressures that might build up because of the inability of individuals or government or business to resolve certain problems. Thus, it is an outlet not only for neighborly instincts but for social action. Voluntarism is often at the leading edge of peaceful change. In this way it tends to stabilize society. And since the movement is self-determining, it cannot flourish except in a free society. Its very existence not only demands, but becomes an important guarantor of, liberty.

There are now more than one million U.S. voluntary hospitals, schools, libraries, orchestras, museums, garden clubs, historical societies, adoption services, drug and alcohol treatment centers, and health associations.

The American Cancer Society is outstanding among these. Started in 1913 by only fifteen men, it approaches its seventy-fifth anniversary as the largest, most influential and most effective private voluntary health organization in history. It is one of those human constructs that support William Faulkner's thesis: people will not merely endure, they will prevail.

The Society came into being with the large purposes of altering the world's beliefs and behavior regarding one of its greatest threats, and revising the dogma and practices of its most learned profession. These coalesced into a single goal: the total control of cancer as a disease of humankind, an objective that seemed almost unattainable at first. But over the past three-quarters of a century, Society programs have helped bring it within striking distance.

The achievement is the sum of the powerful commitment of its millions of volunteers (at present, its volunteer force is 2,500,000 people—more than two of every one hundred U.S. volunteers are American Cancer Society volunteers). Often motivated by a searing experience with cancer, either in themselves or their families or friends, or by their professional concerns (more than fifty thousand U.S. physicians are ACS volunteers), they provide a tenacious force that is not often found even in other kinds of voluntary health organizations.

They represent just about every kind of American in his diverse and pluralistic society: a Boston runner who has lost one leg to bone cancer, and runs coast to coast to raise money for cancer control; a Georgia beauty queen and model who has been unashamed to appear in public to tell of her experience with bowel cancer and a subsequent colostomy. They include an Arizona doctor and one of his patients who organize former cancer patients to help those currently undergoing treatment; a Florida banker who challenges his fellow financiers to match his company's large donation to ACS cancer research; an Atlanta business executive who paints murals in hospital radiology units in many states, so cancer patients won't feel isolated during treatment.

Many ACS volunteers are celebrities—Larry Hagman, Betty Ford, Lena Horne, Happy Rockefeller, Gregory Peck, Raquel Welch, Virginia Graham, and the late John Wayne— but most are obscure, like Mrs. Karen Anderson, who was cured of leukemia as a teenager, married, and has two healthy children of her own.

Former ACS Board chairman and Connecticut judge Charles Ebersol has said that ACS volunteers have one thing in common: "When you move into a new community, I've been told there are two ways to make yourself at home quickly. Contact your church, and get in touch with your local unit of the American Cancer Society. They'll generally be about the finest people in town."

ACS volunteers have shown themselves to be magnanimous, unselfish, and even self-sacrificing, truly their brothers' and sisters' keepers. Yet, strangely, one dimension of their devotion may be measured in actual dollars and cents. Because their work is nearly cost-free (in terms of money), it greatly increases the purchasing power of the donated dollar. The late president Dwight D. Eisenhower estimated that volunteer efforts multiplied the value of monetary gifts by a factor of four; that is, for every dollar given to a well-run, honorable, voluntary organization, the value returned to the public is four dollars.

This has been more than proved by American Cancer Society volunteers. It is not possible to estimate the accrued value of the time and expertise donated by scientists and physicians—all of them recognized leaders in their professions—to the medical and scientific committees of the Society. They give weeks of time to study a mountain of research grant proposals, then fly in from all parts of the country to spend days evaluating them in committee so that the public's money may be put to best use. They also donate their professional judgment on questions of public interest such as carcinogens in the environment. It is equally impossible to put a price on the time of business executives, bankers, students, working women, housewives, children that is donated freely to Society programs of professional education, public education, rehabilitation, support, and service. The Cancer Prevention Studies are monuments to volunteer generosity. Not only were they carried out for a small percent of the cost of professional investigations—saving literally hundreds of millions of dollars—but only dedicated volunteers could have approached near-perfection in multi-year follow-ups of more than a million subjects.

This kind of selfless devotion inspires generosity in others. It has encouraged publishers and broadcasters to donate millions of dollars worth of space and time to ACS lifesaving messages. Thus, the Society has never had to pay for bringing those messages to the public. Similarly, ACS volunteer scientists have evoked the public spirit of congressmen and senators in passing the National Cancer Acts and in supporting the budgets of the National Cancer Institute.

If these and other endeavors, ACS volunteers have helped to save millions of individual lives; and their efforts have resonated throughout the world, helping to create cancer societies in more than a hundred other countries. ACS volunteers have not been merely dedicated, they have been—and continue to be—effective.

Acknowledgments

This project received encouragement and support from many current and retired volunteers and employees of the American Cancer Society. It could not have been written without their help. The author wishes to acknowledge thanks to the following people (in alphabetical order) who gave unstintingly of their time and knowledge to supply information and help and answer questions:

Mr. Lane W. Adams, Dr. Sidney W. Arje, Mr. Stefan Bodnariuk, Dr. Benjamin F. Byrd, Jr., Dr. Charles S. Cameron, Mr. John Mack Carter, Dr. R. Lee Clark, Mr. Alan C. Davis, Mrs. Gerry S. de Harven, Mrs. Helen Del Bove, Hon. Charles R. Ebersol, Dr. Diane Fink, Mr. Emerson Foote, Mr. G. Robert Gadberry, Mr. Lawrence Garfinkel, Dr. E. Cuyler Hammond, Dr. J. Rodney Heller, Mr. Michael F. Heron, Mr. John D. Henry, Dr. Arthur I. Holleb, Dr. Daniel Horn, Mr. John J. Jones, Mrs. Mary Lasker, Dr. John Laszlo, Dr. LaSalle W. Leffall, Jr., Dr. A. Hamblin Letton, Mr. Everett E. Lyle, Mr. Richard P. McGrail, Mr. John Montgomery, Dr. Alfred M. Popma, Dr. Frank R. Rauscher, Mr. Clifton R. Read, Mr. Herbert Seidman, Dr. Michael B. Shimkin, Mr. Edwin Silverberg, Mr. Robert J. Task, Mrs. Francine Timothy, Mr. Thomas W. Ulmer, Mr. Paul Van Nevel, Mr. Francis J. Wilcox, Ms. Genevieve Young.

Special thanks to members of the ACS staff who were helpful beyond the call of duty: Dr. Sourya Henderson and her diligent assistants of the ACS Library, who dug up many obscure documents for reference and volunteered much useful additional information: Ms. Alice Wou of the Library staff who annotated the references and created the index. Thanks, too, to Ms. Diana Perez for a superb job of copy editing; Mr. Ronald Daddea, who managed to find many key ACS materials; Mr. W. Thomas Hellyar, who gave me a copy of the Ph.D. thesis by Dr. Donald F. Shaugnessy of the Society's early history, an invaluable source; and Mr. Michael Back, *fidus Achates*, who was more reliable than the U.S. Post Office. Thanks, too, to Nadia Senchyshyn and Lynn Sleen for unflagging help.

PART ONE

Target: Cancer

I

Halfway to Victory

In 1913 when the American Cancer Society was founded (as the American Society for the Control of Cancer), most physicians and nearly all patients believed that cancer was an incurable disease. Only a handful of doctors, mostly surgeons, rejected this nihilism, based on their experience, but there was no definition of *cure* for the disease, and no cure rate for any tumor. (The generally accepted definition of cancer cure today is no evidence of disease in a patient five years after the start of treatment, and a life expectancy equal to that of someone the same age who has never had cancer.)

At the present time, for all serious tumors—excluding the nearly 100 percent curable skin cancers and *in situ* cancer of the uterine cervix—the relative survival rate of U.S. cancer patients for five years after diagnosis is 49 percent. This takes into account normal life expectancy and includes the risk of dying not only of cancer but of other diseases. The overall cure rate of malignant tumors is probably already higher than that, since current treatments are always being improved and it takes at least five years (because of the five-year survival criterion) to know how effective they are.

In other words, American biomedical science and medicine are about halfway to the goal of controlling cancer in human beings.

Of course, the American Cancer Society is not the only agency responsible for this remarkable progress. But there is little doubt that it was the initiator in organizing the process in the United States, encouraged the participation of others in

3

the attempt, and has played a major role in the achievement. As a result, the Society is one of America's best-known and best-liked organizations. A recent Gallup survey showed that about 95 percent of Americans know its name, and 85 percent approve of what it does. Few institutions of any kind, public or private, have this degree of recognition and acceptance.

Americans back their good opinion of the American Cancer Society with their time, their talents, and their money. More than 2 million volunteers give at least some hours to the Society each year, and many donate days, weeks, even months. Volunteers make Society policies and carry out its programs; they are supported by paid employees at a ratio of 1 to every 650 volunteers.

The Society is supported entirely by private donations. Its fund-raising is done by its volunteers and staff; no professional fund-raising organizations are employed. Reflecting the Society's favorable reputation, gifts are numerous. Although no count is kept of the number of donors, there are probably millions each year. Contributions are generally small, averaging about $10 through mail campaigns and almost certainly less door-to-door, although there are occasional large personal bequests. Because the Society is an independent agency— e.g., not a member of United Way (in recent years, some of its divisions and units have made limited contracts with local chapters of United Way), it receives only about 2 percent of its donations from business or industry.

This extraordinarily broad base of support frees the ACS of obligation to any individual, group, or foundation. It has the liberty to make decisions about controversial subjects guided only by medical and scientific criteria and directed only toward cancer control. Such decisions have not infrequently caused the Society to be attacked by powerful economic and political interests, such as the tobacco industry. The ACS has withstood such assaults because its policies have been carefully pondered and based on reliable evidence.

The Society accepts no money from federal, state, or

local government. Nor does it participate in jointly funded research or other activities with any government agency, although it did so in certain special projects with the federally supported National Cancer Institute in the past. The Society's board of directors and staff are entirely separate from and have no responsibility for National Cancer Institute policies or programs.

Since, the society's endowment revenue is minuscule in relation to the total budget, representing only about .5 percent of annual income, it has been fiscally prudent to budget on the basis of the previous year's receipts. Thus, the ACS budget is based on actual income, which means almost totally on donations received in the previous fiscal year and interest on deposits of that money. For forty years, income has been divided as follows: Sixty percent stays in the fifty-eight separate, incorporated, chartered (generally) statewide divisions of the Society; 25 percent goes to the national research program; 12 percent to run the national office; and 3 percent to medical grants and fellowships. (*Grant* means "grant-in-aid"—a donation for a specific purpose, such as teaching or research, based on a detailed proposal submitted to a jury of the grantee's peers.)

Annual donations to the American Cancer Society have generally outpaced inflation, and have risen through business recessions. In fiscal 1984–85 they totaled about $250 million. More than 80 percent is spent on Society programs, less than 20 percent on administration and fund-raising. It is one of the most efficient of philanthropies.

The American Cancer Society was the first U.S. national voluntary health agency to publish an annual report that includes a full financial statement based on a complete audit by certified public accountants, and the first to give a full accounting of all of its separate divisions.

From its inception, the Society has been jointly organized and run by both lay people and professionals. Its president is always a physician or scientist (except for the first one, Mr. George C. Clark, 1913–1918). Presidents since 1949 have served a single one-year term. The chairman of its board of directors is a lay person, who currently serves for two years. The board of directors, which sets ACS policy, is a fifty-fifty mix of lay and professional people. It averages about 120 members; the fluctuation is due to changes in the number of officer-directors and honorary life members. Because of the size of the board, most policies are suggested by specialized committees whose members are experts in their fields. There are sixty-one committees, subcommittees, and work groups, which may also include non–board members. Their subjects range from audiovisual materials to the worldwide fight against cancer, and take in medicine and science, nursing, childhood cancer, breast cancer, finance, and field services.

The American Cancer Society, Inc., has no official status other than being incorporated under state laws as a private philanthropy, and qualified by the U.S. Treasury Department for tax-free status.

The American Society for the Control of Cancer, founded in 1913, did not become the American Cancer Society until 1945. This apparently small change in nomenclature actually reflected a major reorganization and reorientation. Although the latter Society may be said to have evolved from the former, the modern ACS really began its existence not only under new bylaws but with important additions to and changes in policy and programs in 1945.

Most people when asked what the American Cancer Society does will probably say "Research." That is true, but it is only part of the truth. The only research done by the Society itself is epidemiological—the study of populations' behavior, life habits, work exposures, and other factors in relation to disease. This includes the first large prospective studies on smoking and health and currently the second cancer-prevention study. These surveys are unique.

But the Society also initiated, in 1945, the first nongovernmental national United States program of biomedical research against cancer, by funding accredited investigators, both scientific and clinical, in recognized, responsible institutions across the country. At that time the Society put more money into cancer research than did the federal government. U.S. cancer research has since grown into the largest biomedical research effort in the world.

Once the ACS accepted as its central challenge the control of all human cancer, it began attacking that constellation of diseases at nearly every medical, scientific, and humanistic level.

Society activities and programs rest on a tripartite foundation: research; education; service and rehabilitation.

RESEARCH

Research covers a wide range of scientific and clinical investigations supported by various forms of grants in nearly all leading American medical and scientific institutions and also the large epidemiological surveys done by Society volunteers. Currently, the Society invests more than $70 million a year in funded outside research by either individuals or institutions. Through 1986 its cumulative research expenditure was nearly $900 million.

EDUCATION

The ACS runs a variety of public-education programs designed to alert the public and protect individuals from cancer, and a range of professional-education projects aimed at keeping physicians, nurses, dentists, and various paramedical personnel up-to-date on progress in diagnosis, treatment, and rehabilitation of cancer patients. One program brings physicians from all parts of the world to the United States to learn the latest cancer-management techniques; others include an annual million-dollar donation for clinical fellowships to train young physicians, as well as advanced fellowships to physicians who show promise of becoming outstanding researchers, and oncology (the study of tumors) professorships to improve cancer training of medical students.

SERVICE AND REHABILITATION

ACS service and rehabilitation programs aid cancer patients and their families with rehabilitaiton support by former cancer patients (such as Reach to Recovery for women who have had surgery for breat cancer, and the International Association of Laryngectomees for people who have lost all or part of their larynxes to cancer) counseling for patients and families, loans of sickroom necessities, and patient transportation to physicians' offices or treatment centers. The Society does not operate medical or laboratory facilities, treat patients, or pay doctors' or hospitals' fees. But it does support cancer-detection programs, tissue services—including tumor registries—and the training of cytotechnologists and radiation assistants and pay for certain medications and medically directed and professionally supervised rehabilitation services.

II

Cancer Risk

Cancer is the disease feared most by people throughout the world, and is an abiding health concern of Americans. Much of the fear represents a cultural lag; it is an echo from the time when the disease was largely incurable. Today, cancer is the only one of the four major killing diseases in developed countries that is curable. More than 5 million Americans are alive today who have a history of cancer; more than 3 million were diagnosed as having cancer more than five years ago and most of these will eventually be identified as cured.

These optimistic facts are not cited to minimize cancer's very real threat, but to help redress attitudes to conform with current reality. Cancer is the second leading cause of death in the United States; this year more than 460,000 Americans will die of some form of it, and there will be more than 900,000 new cases. It is estimated that one-third of all babies born in 1987 will eventually develop some type of malignancy during their lifetimes.

While the risk of cancer appears to be mounting in the United States, the largest part of the increase is in lung cancer, which is caused in about 85 percent of cases by smoking cigarettes. The incidence of most other forms of cancer is not rising in this country, in fact most age-adjusted rates for incidence and deaths related to specific sites of cancer are flat or declining. Lung cancer has been the leading cancer cause of death in American men for more than twenty years, and in 1986 it surpassed breast cancer as the leading cause of cancer death in American women. (It was already the leading cause of death in older American women and in all women in twelve states.) Nearly a third of this nation's cancer deaths are caused by tumors in the lung.

Cancer risk in the United States is highest among white males (more than one in three develop cancer), slightly lower among black males, and lower for white women and black women, in that order. Although cancer kills more American children between the ages of three and fourteen than any other malady, fewer than 1 percent of cancers occur in children. It is primarily a disease of old age. And since Americans now sucumb much less frequently to other diseases or causes in middle age, the population of the country is growing older—hence the cancer risk is rising. According to Herbert Seidman, ACS assistant vice-president for epidemiology and statistics, "Among American men, cancer of the prostate has come to equal lung cancer as the leading long-term cancer threat."

WHAT CANCER IS

Although *cancer* is a singular noun, it is generally taken to mean not a single disease but a constellation of more than a hundred types of tumors with certain common characteristics. Cancer cells derive from normal cells by a process called "carcinogenesis," which gives them the ability to create new growth (neoplasia). They are often simplified, more primitive versions of normal cells, but, unlike normal cells, they have the capacity for unlimited growth. They do not necessarily grow faster than normal cells, but they never stop growing or dividing via the process known as mitosis. Thus, unlike normal cells, which have a finite number of divisions built into their genetic code, they are immortal.

They also take priority over normal cells, stealing their nourishment and thereby starving the body and causing the wasting away (cachexia and anemia) often seen in patients with advanced cancer. They continue to replicate *ad infinitum* unless arrested by therapy or until they kill the host.

Cancers tend to begin on the outer or inner surfaces of organs or in their ducts or vessels and to mimic the normal cells of these organs, even often secreting hormones if they are of glandular origin. They may begin as single cells, which divide into two, four, eight cells in endless geometric progression. In certain organs, cancer cells can be detected before they become a visible (without a microscope) or palpable tumor; at this stage they are called "cancer *in situ*" and can be removed. Thus, cancer can in effect be prevented if cancer cells are detected early enough. (There is an unresolved semantic debate as to whether cancer *in situ* is truly cancer; which leads to a further debate as to whether finding and removing the abnormal cells at this early stage is preventive, or merely seems to prolong life by intervening earlier in an inexorable pathological process.) Finding and removing cancer *in situ* occurs most frequently in the cervix, for which there is a reliable cancer-cell test known as the Pap test and in the large bowel, or colon, where cancer usually starts in, and is at first confined to, a polyp.

Cancer cells at most sites are not usually detected *in situ*, however. They continue growing silently, giving no evidence of their presence, until they form a tumor. A tumor, in its early stages, does not generally cause pain or other symptoms, and is considered most curable at this time—although even a small tumor may occasionally be fatal if it disrupts the functioning of a vital organ. If undetected, the tumor continues to grow. Most create "stromas"—supporting networks of connective tissue and blood vessels. These are made of normal cells. Thus, the invading cancer not only steals nourishment from normal cells but also co-opts them to serve its malignant metabolic needs, bringing oxygen and nourishment, carrying off waste, it enslaves them in their own destruction.

Cancers can penetrate biological barriers that stop normal tissue or benign tumors (cartilage and tendons are obstacles to cancers' growth, but bone is not) and eventually spread through invasion into adjacent structures. At the leading edge of invading tumors there is usually a band of lymphoid cells, evidence that the body is attempting to defend its integrity through its immune system. Cancer at this stage is called "invasive," but may still be localized and controllable.

However, the longer cancer persists, the more menacing it becomes. This is so because of the unique ability of malignant cells not merely to penetrate adjacent organs but to break off from the orginal tumor when it has reached a certain size, and to remain viable while voyaging through the lymphatic or blood circulatory system to other parts of the body. There they colonize and continue to grow. This process is known as metastasis. Different tumors differ in the likelihood and swiftness of metastasis.

At first the spread may be regional, the cancer cells trapped by lymph nodes in a certain region of the body. Treatment is more likely to be successful at this point than later, for eventually these migrating cells will escape from the region and form multiple tumors in other, more distant organs. At this late stage it may be impossible to cure the patient. Most cancer deaths are caused by metastasis.

TREATING CANCER

Four methods are used to treat cancer, alone or in various combinations: surgery; radiation therapy; chemotherapy (the use of anticancer drugs to exploit differences between certain cancer cells and normal cells); and immunotherapy (supporting or strengthening the body's immune system, which may not always be able to repel cancer cells unaided). Immunotherapy is still considered an experimental form of treatment.

There are also supportive measures, such as hyperalimentation—infusing a complete liquid diet through a vein to compensate for cancer's nutritional thievery—and the use of transfusions of whole or fractions of blood. Not curative in themselves, these measures buy time for patients, allowing other treatments to take effect.

PREVENTING CANCER

Cancer is preventable. Although the precise etiology or origin of the disease is still unknown, many proximate causes have been identified—that is, substances or behaviors that result in cancer.

In the history of medicine, it has not been necessary to identify the cause or understand the entire process of a disease in order to prevent it. A classic example is the case of the London physician John Snow, who in early September 1849 saw a violent cholera epidemic—"the most terrible which ever occurred in this kingdom. . . . I suspected some contamination of the water of the much-frequented street pump in Broad Street," Dr. Snow reported later. He looked at the water "with the naked eye" and saw some "white, flocculant particles." Investigating eighty-nine deaths, "I found that nearly all had taken place within a short distance of the pump." Others might be connected with the pump through water sold in chemists' shops, public houses, and by some people's preference for the Broad Street water, although they lived a few streets away.

"I had an interview with the Board of Guardians of St. James's parish and represented the above circumstances. In consequence, the handle of the pump was removed on the following day."

That ended the epidemic. Later, Dr. Snow, who is credited as a pioneer in suggesting that disease might be waterborne, showed that the Broad Street well was contaminated by sewage. Dr. Snow's research is an early example of epidemiology leading to the prevention of disease and death. The actual cause of cholera, a type of bacillus known as *Vibrio cholerae*, was not identified until thirty-five years later, in 1884.

The earliest known "cause" of cancer was found in 1775 by Sir Percivall Pott, a British surgeon. Pott noticed that chimney sweeps had a high incidence of scrotal cancer. He deduced that this came from soot lodged in the folds of the scrotum. Chimney sweeps did not have adequate bathing facilities; Dr. Pott suggested that they might avoid scrotal cancer by bathing more frequently and more carefully.

It was not until more than a century later that the carcinogenic element in soot—benzo-a-pyrene—was discovered. This same substance is found in many kinds of smoke, including tobacco smoke. It is thought to be one of the causes of the high incidence of lung cancer among cigarette smokers.

Other causes of cancer are overexposure of light-skinned people to sunlight, overexposure to ionizing radiation (X ray and other forms), inhaling uranium dust, inhaling asbestos particles, and high workplace exposure without adequate protection to certain chemicals used in dyes, pesticides, plastics, and other products. Although it is popularly supposed that we are swimming in a sea of carcinogens, and that these are causing most of our cancers, the truth is that chemically induced cancers are generally confined to the workplace, and all known workplace carcinogens are related to only a small proportion—about 5 to 8 percent—of cancers in this country. By far the greatest number of lethal tumors in the United States whose source is known are caused by smoking tobacco.

III

Organizing the Attack

Cancer is unique among the major killing diseases: "In no other does the patient bear so large a share of responsibility for recognizing the subtle first signs . . . and for realizing that they are worth investigating, for in no other disease of comparable seriousness do the first warning signs seem so trivial. In no other does the patient alone influence the outcome to so great a degree," wrote Dr. Charles S. Cameron.

These facts are an important part of the reason for the founding and growth of the American Cancer Society. If a condition is perceived as hopeless or incurable, then it becomes pointless for doctors to diagnose or treat it, or for patients to take the responsibility of seeking diagnosis or therapy. Thus, in 1913, when the American Society for the Control of Cancer was founded, fatalism was an accomplice in the remorseless progression of cancer. The ten physicians who helped found the Society believed that popular and professional fear of cancer should be eradicated. For the disease was being cured in 1913, and long before that.

As early as Byzantium, around A.D. 500–600, surgeons had begun to abandon the therapeutic nihilism toward the disease—e.g., that no treatment could cure cancer—established by Egyptian physicians in the Smith and Ebers Papyruses some 4,000 years earlier. Aetios of Amida (A.D. 527–565) wrote a medical encyclopedia containing detailed directions for mastectomy (surgical breast removal) to treat breast cancer, and a careful description of cancer of the uterus. Other Byzantine doctors boldly removed tumors of

15

the skin, lip, and other external body parts with the purpose of curing patients. Surgery had come a long way by 1913, and the discovery of ionizing radiation (X ray) in 1895 had provided a means of diagnosing tumors within the body as well as a new modality of treatment, although it was not widely used for that purpose when the ASCC was founded.

In the mid–nineteenth century, a German surgeon, Christian Albert Theodor Billroth, had performed a variety of operations for cancers of the esophagus, larynx, stomach, breast, and intestine. He followed up 548 patients, and among the 170 operated on for breast cancer, found a three-year survival rate of 4.7 percent. The first successful operation for a tumor of the spinal cord had been performed in Britain by Sir Victor Horsley long before the American Society for the Control of Cancer began; and Dr. William S. Halsted of Johns Hopkins University had perfected the "Halsted radical" operation for removing a cancerous breast, together with a good deal of other tissue, in 1891.

Thus some of those at the (literally) cutting edge of medicine, the most aggressive and experimental surgeons, were curing some cancers. The gynecologists who helped found the Society for the Control of Cancer believed with Dr. Howard C. Taylor, Sr., that "if we had seen the cases [of uterine cancer] at an earlier stage of the disease we could probably have cured some of the patients."

This was almost certainly a minority opinion among gynecologists and in the medical profession as a whole. As one example, Dr. J. E. Janvrin, a former president of the American Gynecological Society, had told his colleagues in 1903 regarding cancer of the cervix, then the leading cause of cancer death among American women, "In view of how little can be accomplished by surgery one is often led to think that perhaps it might be best not to attempt any radical measures in the treatment of this disease but merely to attempt to prolong life and make it more endurable." A British physician, Sir John Bland-Sutton, later recalled, "We used to hold consultations as to whether an operation was justifiable or not. If there was any doubt, all consultants advised waiting until the lymph glands became involved." In other words, until the case became hopeless.

A first step toward curing more cancer would seem to have been educating the medical professional to be more aggressive in diagnosing and treating it. And this was certainly discussed by leaders in medicine—in the American Medical Association, the American Congress of Physicians and Surgeons, and the American Gynecological Society. They had been addressed by Dr. Livingston Farrand, the executive secretary of the National Organization for the Study and Prevention of Tuberculosis, then the only United States group attempting to educate the public about a killing disease. Dr. Farrand had pointed out, "You cannot get a number of physicians who are competent to make an early diagnosis of tuberculosis. And when it comes to cancer in the average community, the failure on the part of the average physician, and even the average surgeon, is shocking." Dr. Farrand had said that they had that problem to deal with, as well as educating "the laity."

Yet the founders of the ASCC did not choose professional education as their initial priority. In fact the ASCC's founders deliberately avoided professional education because they felt that it would be "impolitic" and "might tend to discourage the cooperation of the medical profession."

Instead the Society decided that the best way to change medical opinion and practice was to go over the heads of professionals and appeal to the public. It encouraged people to seek early diagnosis so that the disease (if present) might be found at a more manageable stage, and sought to overcome the popular fear of cancer so that people would not assume it was incurable but would demand treatment.

There was some indication that the public wanted, or might accept, cancer education. In 1891 a German gynecologist, Dr. Georg Winter, had begun urging that women be informed about symptoms of uterine cancer so that they would seek prompt treatment. Dr. Howard C. Taylor, one of the ASCC founders, recalled later that "Dr. Winter, in Königsberg in East Prussia, did some educational work through the midwives in that city. This is the first lay educational work in cancer of which I have any knowledge."

It is probable that Winter's efforts impressed organized American medicine. According to Dr. Taylor, "In 1905 when Dr. Lewis McMurtry was president of the American Medical Association, he appointed Dr. John Clark and Dr. Frank Simpson to investigate the cancer problem. About this time a committee headed by Dr. Thomas Cullen was appointed by the College of Surgeons to work along the same line. . . . It was a paper read by Dr. Frederick L. Hoffman on May 7, 1913, at a meeting of the American Gynecological Society that crystallized the subject and led to the formation of the American Society for the Control of Cancer."

If the Society would succeed, it first had to take cancer out of the closet. In 1913 the disease was not named in polite society. Patients were routinely shielded from knowing that they had a malignancy. The patient's family might be told, but they were unlikely to discuss this even with their closest friends; it was shameful to have a relative with cancer. The seventh leading cause of death in the United States at that time, responsible for some 75,000 deaths per year, cancer was not mentioned in newspaper obituaries. The standard euphemism was "a long illness." It ranked in shame with syphillis and other unmentionable afflictions.

In 1906 a British physician, Dr. C. P. Childe, wrote the first book to inform the public about cancer. He called it *The Control of a Scourge*. Only the subtitle contained the word *cancer*. Not until 1926 would it be issued as *Cancer and the Public*.

In the 1913 climate of cancer phobia, it took great editorial courage to do what the *Ladies' Home Journal* did the month that the Society was founded: publish an article by the well-known journalist Samuel Hopkins Adams with the inflammatory title "What Can We Do About Cancer?" According to Dr. Taylor, this article was inspired by the committee of the American College of Surgeons, appointed to study the cancer problem. Dr. Cullen, head of the committee, who also became a founder of the ASCC, endorsed the piece.

The Adams article had impact simply because it discussed a taboo subject in lay language for a mass audience. The information it conveyed was primitive by today's standards, reflecting the state of medical knowledge at the time. Adams concluded with several "truths." One was that cancer usually develops from continued irritation. Another was that "if the irritation can be removed, the cancer can be averted." Statements like these were not far advanced over those of the doctors of Byzantium. But Adams's third point while not totally accurate, was most important: "If the development of cancer be determined in the early stages, the patient can probably be cured by operation, but not by any other method." (Actually, a Chicago woman had been treated for breast cancer by X ray as early as 1896, and an epithelioma of the cheek had been reported cured in Sweden by this means by Dr. T.A.U. Sjorgen in 1899.)

While the public was being exposed to an unvarnished discussion of the unmentionable, ASCC founders were lining up powerful medical support. In 1913 both the Clinical Congress of Surgeons of North America, and the American Medical Association endorsed the Cancer Society. The AMA House of Delegates unanimously resolved "that this movement deserves the cooperation of the medical profession, and the Association heartily commends its worthy purpose."

Once establishd, the ASCC began to change the climate of cancer. And as its activities were successful, they led to policies and programs that were seminal to the Society's future, right up until today.

The organization established a printing program that started with *Campaign Notes*, a monthly bulletin. Insurance companies were inspired to seek Society help in preparing materials for their policyholders; and later, urged on by the ASCC, the director of the U.S. Census Bureau, W. J. Harris, prepared and published the first national U.S. cancer-mortality statistics. North Dakota's state legislature passed a law requiring their state laboratory director to make free microscopic examinations of suspected cancer tissues removed during surgery. Nearly all state boards of health east of the Mississippi endorsed the ASCC within its first two years.

In his history of the Society, Donald E. Shaughnessy states that "Dr. F. C. Wood reported that 'because of this publicity, patients were presenting themselves earlier.' " And several state boards of health found the same thing. In fact, Dr. F. L. Hoffman of the ASCC stated that by 1916, cancer deaths had decreased "in places where the Society has been most active."

On the other hand, the medical profession had not reacted as hoped. Many doctors remained more frightened and pessimistic about the disease than their patients. Dr. Edward Reynolds, head of the ASCC's committee on organization, blamed a number of cases of delayed diagnosis and treatment on his fellow practitioners and opined that "this condition can only be improved by raising the standards of medical schools and the state requirements for admission to practice. Writing articles in medical journals seems useless because the doctors whom it is most necessary to reach do not read them."

The ASCC needed money to operate. At first the executive committee thought that $10,000 a year would cover their expenses, but since they were all busy teaching and practicing medicine, they did not have much time for fund-raising. One of the men given most credit for starting the Society, Dr. Clement Cleveland, was able to help by proxy. His daughter, Mrs. Robert G. (Elsie) Mead, was active in women's clubs and charity and community work. Mrs. Mead took on the job of raising money for the new organization and was later made chairman of the Finance Committee. This established another precedent, considerably more revolutionary in that day than this: equal opportunity and status for women in the Society.

Elsie Mead was by all accounts a dynamic person who used her social connections to further good causes. Thomas Debevoise, her husband's law partner, was brought into the organization by Mrs. Mead, as were the other four layfounders at the Harvard Club meeting: Messrs. Clark, Lamont, Macy, and Parsons.

Mrs. Mead started by proposing different levels of membership—"patron," "benefactor," and so on—with an appropriate scale of contribution. Standard membership was $5 a year; there were 394 such contributors by 1915. But the primary goal was never just money; it was explicitly stated that the membership be as broad as possible to include volunteers who would be active in the Society. That year's budget of $6,997 included $4,888 for salaries, $354 for rent, and $75 for telephone and telegraph.

The executive committee decided that since membership fees were not meeting current expenses, the ASCC needed a more stable financial underpinning. They asked for $15,000. Mrs. Mead got fifteen pledges of $1,000 each in the thirty days from November 8 to December 8, 1915. She was voted "a unanimous hearty vote of thanks." Three years later the Society's bulletin noted that Elsie Mead, "more than anyone else is responsible for the financial planning which has made possible the organization and continuance of the Society for the Control of Cancer."

Within months of the Society's founding, various local cancer groups were being formed. This new factor forced the ASCC's hand. The founders had considered the possibility of local chapters when the group was started, but had decided that while these would be valuable and should be affiliated with the national organization, "efforts should be first directed to perfecting the national organization and securing membership therein." Now they had to face the question: Would a plethora of local cancer organizations fragment and perhaps frustrate the ASCC's drive toward national cancer control? Dr. James Reynolds warned that this could happen. "The institution of a multiplicity of independent and often conflicting organizations is always a misfortune to the purpose for which they are organized," he said. His committee on organization voted that local groups be organized and given status within the ASCC, but was voted down. However, the pressure created by the growing number of local career organizations forced the ASCC to consider creating state committees.

In 1916 the Society began to appoint leading physicians to form committees in their given states. As an example, Dr. Wiliam J. Mayo, the senior Mayo brother, was selected as state chairman of the Minnesota chapter of the ASCC. Individual physicians rather than state medical societies were preferred as the initiators of state and local chapters because the leaders of the ASCC insisted on involving lay people in cancer control from the start. In this decision they showed uncanny prescience. Lay people gave powerful help in directing the ASCC toward its goal of helping lay people protect themselves against cancer. A similar pattern has been followed by other disease-fighting organizations that started later; they have proved most effective when incorporating the model of professional/lay cooperation created by the founders of the ASCC.

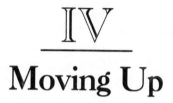

IV

Moving Up

By April 1922 the ASCC had the framework of a national organization; there were nuclei in forty-eight states, Hawaii, the Philippines, and ten Canadian provinces as well. But it was controlled by physicians, most of whom were in the Northeast, and this was where about three-quarters of the Society's funds were raised.

The ASCC's modest expansion had taken place under President Charles A. Powers, elected in 1919. A New York surgeon who had been forced to move to Denver after recovering from tuberculosis, Dr. Powers set three axioms for the Society's public-education activities:

1. Cancer is at first a local disease.
2. With early recognition and prompt treatment, the patient's life can often be saved.
3. Through ignorance and delay, thousands of lives are needlessly sacrificed.

The Society's printed materials, designed to educate the public, listed the following danger signals that may mean cancer:

- Any lump, especially in the breast
- Any irregular bleeding or discharge
- Any sore that does not heal, particularly about the tongue, mouth, or lips
- Persistent indigestion with loss of weight

Dr. J. E. Rush was hired by the ASCC to fill the newly created post of field director in 1922. His job was to travel around the country and involve physicians in cancer control. He reported that where doctors were not active against cancer, it was because they hadn't been briefed on the Society's program. Once informed, they were usually cooperative.

This, and other missionary work, required more money. Mrs. Mead, who had gone to France for the Red Cross during the World War, had returned to her ASCC work in the United States and recruited more members. She wrote 2,000 letters to people listed in the New York *Social Register*, and got nearly 600 recruits, most of whom paid considerably more than the $5 membership fee. The Society's budget was more than $60,000 in 1922.

It was not easy to reach a consensus on how to approach the sticky tasks of educating doctors without seeming to insult them, and how to educate the public about cancer without creating cancerphobia. The *Journal of the American Medical Association* editorialized in 1921 that "an inevitable accompaniment of directing special attention to any disease is to arouse in a certain number of persons phobias almost as terrifying as the disease feared," and went on to criticize some of the "danger signals" as "capable of shattering even a normal mentality."

In 1923 the Society hired its first managing director, Dr. George A. Soper. An epidemiologist who had helped track down the famous "Typhoid Mary," Dr. Soper was the first nonsurgeon to wield authority in the ASCC. He was also an iconoclast, even more critical of the organization than was the *JAMA*. "It is questionable," he said, "whether the optimistic attitude [that ASCC materials for patients emphasized] furnishes the strongest motive force which it is practicable to employ." He stirred debate about the Society's basic approach: Should it be relentlessly optimistic, or could people be motivated more effectively through fear?

Soper was an activist who appeared to seek confrontations. He found the Society's printed materials out-of-date, filled with statements that "it would be difficult to substantiate." The Society had begun to hold annual national cancer weeks, starting October 30 to November 5, 1921. A highlight of that event was the first radio address on cancer, a fifteen-minute speech by ASCC president Dr. Powers. Dr. Soper criticized such "spasmodic efforts to rouse the public."

But he had positive ideas and programs to offer as well, and set the agenda for the Society for the next ten years in an outline of "Principles and Policies" presented to the executive committee in December 1923. As an epidemiologist, he was conscious of the lack of statistics on cancer incidence and mortality, which were essential in giving direction to programs of cancer control. His first point was, therefore, that the Society ought to be developing its information-gathering function. He also insisted on accuracy of statement in ASCC materials and the use of fear as a motive force. In addition, he wanted the organization to encourage the establishment of cancer clinics and cancer institutes.

Soper's suggestions were generally supported by the eminent Dr. James Ewing, although Dr. Ewing also passed along some demurrers he had heard, and with which he at least partly agreed: Ewing said there was "too much assurance that surgery is the only safe method," and there had been "false statements about the limitations and dangers of radiation."

Thomas Debevoise offered some constructive criticism of his own: "There must be some middle ground between too much hope and too much horror," he wrote to Soper. "Care must be taken to [tie] hope to prompt action and horror to delay." He also offered a more diplomatic approach to physician education: "It is suggested that the Society should 'instruct' the medical men. [But] we should avoid giving general practitioners the idea that we think they need instruction. [Can't we say that a Society purpose] is to help medical men be properly informed in regard to the latest thought on the cancer question?"

In 1926 there were 800 venereal clinics, more than 600

tuberculosis clinics, and more than 100 heart clinics, but almost no clinics that specialized in cancer. Although several cancer clinics and cancer hospitals had been founded early in the century, all of them were in New York. By 1927–28, only five other states—Pennsylvania, Michigan, Minnesota, Colorado, Ohio—and the District of Columbia had cancer clinics or hospitals.

More cancer clinics were needed because so many patients were not getting the best available diagnosis and treatment in general hospitals or from private physicians. Wrote Dr. Byron B. Davis of Omaha, Nebraska: "There must be no superficial examinations, no time-consuming hesitation, no trifling with a possibly early malignancy, no admonition to 'wait and see what develops.' "

Supporting cancer clinics became a major project of the Society. However, in pushing for specialized treatment centers, the ASCC had to avoid alienating doctors. The Society balanced support for clinics with the stipulation that there was no intention to interfere in the private practice of medicine.

But it had created the vector for change, by focusing on cancer as a public health problem. The more the public became aware of the possibility of cure, the greater their demand for proper diagnosis and state-of-the-art therapy.

In 1926 the Massachusetts legislature passed a law intended, among other things, "to promote the prevention and cure of cancer." Under this statute the Department of Public Health was authorized to transform the Norfolk state hospital into a cancer clinic, and to buy $70,000 worth of radium for the facility. The department was also authorized to establish other cancer clinics in the state, "with or without the cooperation of the local medical profession."

The Society kept pushing for more such state-owned facilities, and for making cancer as much a responsibility of public health departments as tuberculosis was at the time. Clinics and education were effective. The Pennsylvania State Cancer Commission had surveyed patients and physicians in

1923, and compared the findings with a 1913 survey. "People are applying more promptly than they used," reported J. M. Wainwright, chairman of the commission. "The period of delay between the first symptom and the operation has been reduced from 14 to 8 months in the ten-year period. It was also discovered that physicians were applying the proper treatment in a shorter period of time. . . . The delay from the first consultation to the operation had been cut from 12 to 3.9 months."

However, other states were lagging. A personal survey of the West in 1927 by Dr. Raymond Brokaw, field representative of the ASCC, yielded many negative reports:

TEXAS: No cancer hospitals or clinics.

NEW MEXICO: Deaths not classified: no county or state hospitals. Not practical to organize the ASCC in this state.

WASHINGTON STATE: State chairman resigned, out of sympathy with Society methods, believes "undue alarm being created in minds of laity."

MONTANA: No cancer clinics or special facilities. Cancer death rate rose from 40 per 1,000 in 1910 to 79 in 1926.

A Society survey in 1928 revealed that there were only 72 grams of radium in fewer than 400 hospitals in the whole of the United States, and 526 X-ray machines. There were only 40 diagnostic clinics, most of them in Massachusetts and New York. In 1929 the country counted about 125,000 cancer deaths.

V

Pullback and Advance

In 1928 the board of director's of the ASCC asked for Dr. Soper's resignation, and accepted it with several encomiums for the work he had done. He was replaced in 1929 by Dr. Clarence Cook Little, a scientist (genetics), teacher (pathology), and administrator (past president of the University of Maine and then the University of Michigan, from which he resigned to join the ASCC). Dr. Little was and continued to be director of the Roscoe B. Jackson Memorial Laboratories in Bar Harbor, Maine, while director of the ASCC; for sixteen years he commuted between the two jobs.

Dr. Clarence Cook Little was a powerful personality who set new directions for the Society during his tenure, which lasted until 1944. Independent but not undiplomatic, he was an excellent ambassador for the ASCC, and an optimist primarily interested in research and therapy. In 1930, after familiarizing himself with the workings of the Society, Dr. Little went to Europe to make a personal survey of the medical and scientific state of cancer from Edinburgh to Warsaw. Reporting to the ASCC board of directors, he noted that European professionals were almost unanimously opposed to lay education in cancer, because they feared it would give rise to cancer phobia—that persistent bugaboo among physicians on both sides of the Atlantic. Instead, they emphasized experimentation and research.

Little was obviously sympathetic to the European viewpoint. Without adequate treatment and research facilities, he told the ASCC board, "a superficial program of lay publicity" would only lead more patients to cancer phobia, quacks, and disillusionment, and ultimately create antagonism against the organization.

The board followed his lead. Little divided the United States into four regions and hired four physicians to bring the Society's message of cancer control to their colleagues in each region. During the next five years, the ASCC concentrated on professional education: sending exhibits and speakers to medical meetings, publishing and distributing professional literature, and giving lectures at medical schools. The push for cancer clinics went on; the American College of Surgeons cooperated in seeing that more such facilities met Society standards. The organization also kept a running inventory of the services and equipment available at the clinics.

Dr. Little's program worked to his and the board's satisfaction. By 1932 he was authorized to approach the general Federation of Women's Clubs to enlist their members in a public-education campaign. The clubwomen were receptive. By 1935 he had completely reversed his position: "Existing facilities are entirely adequate to care for many more cancer cases than are now availing themselves of the opportunity of early diagnosis and treatment," he reported. "Lay education had lagged far behind." Now was the time for a "widespread and intensive campaign" to inform the public about "the prevention of cancer."

Dr. Little's early years with the Society unfortunately coincided with the stock-market crash of 1929 and the Great Depression. No institution was immune to the resulting economic and social upheaval. For the Society it meant a drop in income, leading to staff cuts and salary reductions. It decimated private medical practice, forcing successful physicians to augment their incomes with other work—leaving less time for volunteer Society activities. Plans for new cancer clinics were scrapped for lack of funds. And to fill the vacuum left by diminished philanthrophy and the shortcomings and, failures of private enterprise, the government was pressured to take over and initiate a great many programs in health and welfare.

There was also a thrust toward government-insured medical treatment for all. Many doctors suspected this would lead to socialized medicine, and thus became wary of any philanthropic enterprise that dealt with public health. "The profession is inclined to view with a good deal of antagonism national organizations which have as their objective the education of the laity," Dr. Little reported to the ASCC board in 1934.

In 1937 President Franklin D. Roosevelt signed the National Cancer Institute Act, to "provide for and to foster the continuous study of the cause, the prevention, the diagnosis and the treatment of cancer." It called for a six-member National Advisory Council; the first council included four of the ASCC's directors. Congress appropriated $750,000 to build and equip a National Cancer Institute (NCI) in Bethesda, Maryland, and another $400,000 for the first year's operating expenses (half was earmarked for buying radium). The institute was mainly research-oriented, creating fellowships and publishing its own journal.

The Society's need for more volunteers to carry out public education, and for new sources of money, forced it to broaden its volunteer base. The ASCC Executive Committee decided that women would make the best public-education volunteers for a number of reasons: The campaign would go into people's homes, where tact and patience would be essential; it would require a good deal of time, which many women could more easily spare in the mid-1930s than could their husbands; and the emphasis would be on cancers that affected women.

Mrs. Marjorie G. Illig, chairman of the General Federation of Women's Clubs Committee on Public Health was appointed lay field representative of the ASCC in 1936. With her help, Dr. Little prepared a proposal to involve clubwomen in the Society. The concept was that of an army—The

Women's Field Army—with an army's discipline, vertical organization, officer corps, and foot volunteers. Members even wore brown uniforms with insignia of rank. "When the dead and dying from cancer," wrote Dr. Herman Crowell, "are regarded in a similar light to the slain and wounded on the field of battle, somewhat the same compulsion that leads to victory against an invading army will operate in the struggle to vanquish this disease."

The Women's Field Army (WFA) was a quantum leap forward in volunteer power. "In 1935 there were fifteen thousand people active in cancer control throughout the United States," wrote Dr. Little in 1939. "At the close of 1938, there were ten times that number. This growth has been due solely to the Women's Field Army."

In numbers there were wealth and strength. For the first time since the stock-market crash, the Society's annual budget topped $100,000. Thirty percent of the money went to the National Society to pay for literature, films, etc., and the other 70 percent to the Field Army for their expenses.

Years of public and professional cancer education by the men of the ASCC had made "inroads . . . on the prejudices against the use of the word *cancer*, but the larger part of the public remained unconvinced that cancer could be cured . . . and many men in the profession were skeptical of the value of lay education." The majority of doctors were as unconvinced about cancer's curability as their patients.

The Women's Field Army held "tag days" to raise money and build optimism. They started subsidizing needy cancer patients' travel to diagnostic and treatment centers, under medical supervision, and encouraged public and private donations to hospitals, clinics, and laboratories. A congresswoman, Mrs. Edith Nourse Rogers of Massachusetts, who was also a member of the WFA, introduced a bill that Congress adopted, calling on President Roosevelt to proclaim April of each year National Cancer Control Month. Every president since Roosevelt has done this.

The irresistible expansion of Society activities through the WFA forced the board to rethink its priorities and broaden the Society's articles of incorporation "to organize and administer the WFA, to aid voluntarily, in cooperation with accredited physicians, indigent cancer patients in securing adequate diagnosis or treatment; to assist, voluntarily, in the establishment, development, equipment, or maintenance of hospitals, clinics, laboratories, or other facilities for the care of cancer patients; and generally to carry on any other activities which may contribute toward the control of cancer, except the actual treatment of cancer patients or the actual operation of hospitals, clinics, laboratories, or other facilities for such treatment."

The WFA grew to about 700,000 officers and troops, aided in no small part by the support of successive presidents of the Federation of Women's Clubs: Mmes. G. M. Reynolds, R. C. Lawson and S. O. Dunbar. The army grew even during World War II, when many of its members took on other volunteer duties to serve the war effort.

VI

Transformation

In 1943 my housekeeper was diagnosed as having cancer of the uterus, and the doctors said that nothing could be done. I was shocked. I learned that there was practically no research. I went to the American Cancer Society, which was then the American Society to Control Cancer, and found that the Women's Field Army was raising about two hundred and forty thousand dollars a year. The Society was doing nothing about research. There wasn't enough money. It was run by doctors, and they knew very little about fund-raising or publicity. I talked to Dr. Little, and suggested that they try to get the message about cancer control to more people, on the radio, which was then the major broadcast medium. He said that there was no way to do this, the word *cancer* couldn't be mentioned on the air.

I spoke to my husband, Albert, who was president of an advertising agency [Lord & Thomas], and said we needed to reach the public via radio but the word *cancer* was unmentionable on radio. His brother had died of cancer. He called Niles Trammell, the president of NBC, and told him of this situation. Trammell called Dave Sarnoff, the head of RCA, who owned NBC, and pretty soon the way was opened. Two of the most popular network shows were comedies. "Fibber McGee and Molly" and "Bob Hope." Both gave serious messages about the need for money to do cancer research. And the checks poured into the Society, so many they had to send the envelopes to a bank and have the tellers open them.

—Interview with Mrs. Albert D. (Mary) Lasker, October 23, 1984

During his sixteen years with the Society, Dr. Little worked to expand its board of directors, to increase the

33

number of lay people on it, and to create a truly national organization. The year before he arrived, the board was expanded from five to thirty members, but only three came from west of the Allegheny Mountains, and one-third of the members were New Yorkers. During the 1930s, Little campaigned for a larger and more representative group: "A board of thirty is too large for repeated intimate meetings and too small to give anything like adequate national representation.

The directors promised to consider doubling their number at the 1939 annual meeting. But they were reluctant to do what Dr. Little was asking: elect a majority of lay members. Most of the directors were physicians, and they viewed cancer as primarily a medical problem to be dealt with by professionals. Indeed, many had been opposed to creating the Women's Field Army, because they foresaw the possibility of lay dominance: they had accepted the WFA only after assurance that it would be under constant supervision.

The Field Army's success and growth created even more pressures for change. Little began campaigning for a complete reorganization. In 1941 he warned, "There is an increasing pressure being brought upon the Society by the rapidly increasing thousands [of patients] who have absorbed the information and are applying it. They wish us to assume the responsibility of completing the process, for completed it must be, if not under our guidance, then under someone else's."

In other words, if the doctors wouldn't share power, they stood a good chance of losing it to some other cancer-control organization.

Dr. Little had long believed that education and treatment were not enough. "The conquest of cancer will not be complete," he wrote in 1943, "unless and until the nature of the disease and the circumstances of its origin are understood. We are at present at an interesting and important crisis. At a time when the shores of a whole continent of problems in cancer research are clearly visible to the investigator, various factors are present which temporarily postpone and may even prevent our landing."

In 1944 a concerned Mary Lasker read an article by Dr. Cornelius P. Rhoads, the distinguished cancer specialist of Memorial Hospital. Dr. Rhoads said that if any research institution could have a budget of a half-million dollars a year for cancer investigations, they would certainly make progress toward finding a cure. Mrs. Lasker was "infuriated when I read that there was no single place which had as much as five hundred thousand dollars for cancer research. . . . That wouldn't even be a suitable sum for an advertising campaign for a toothpaste." She asked Dr. Little how much the Society was spending on research. When she learned that the Society had no research program, she was stunned. She again went to her husband, one of the leading advertising men in the United States. Albert Lasker was sympathetic, but could give little time. Instead he delegated a young associate, Emerson Foote, both of whose parents had died of cancer.

Mr. Foote talked to Dr. Little and assured him that if the Society ran a professional fund-raising campaign, it could easily raise $5 million to finance cancer research. At the same time, a committee of doctors appointed by Little to study Society problems came up with a plan for a board of directors "scattered over the nation and deeply concerned with cancer control."

Little combined Foote's ideas with those of his committee and recommended a governing board for the national Society. This board would include leading men and women from law, labor, education, industry, government, banking, and business. Through such people, the Society's program would reach labor unions, colleges, business offices, and factories. The Society's directors feared that this new board might seize control, but Little reassured them that the bylaws would prevent this. They approved the governing board.

In 1944 Foote and the Laskers persuaded the Society to hire Lee Casey, a public-relations expert and fund-raiser, and the Laskers offered to pay half his salary. Casey brought in Eric Johnston, a very well-known and well-liked business leader and president of the United States Chamber of Commerce, as volunteer chairman of the next year's (1945) campaign with the approval of Society president Dr. Frank Adair.

In July 1944 Mrs. Lasker received a donation from Raymond Loewy Associates, the design firm, and forwarded it to Dr. Adair with a note: "I got this money from Mr. Loewy on the basis that the Society wished to have a research fund for the investigation and research in treatments and cures in fields other than surgery, X-ray, and radium—in other words, for research in chemotherapy." In another letter she added, "The important thing is that a research policy be established promptly so that research in the field of cancer be coordinated and directed rather than continue as in the past to be scattered and disorganized." Dr. Adair responded that the Society had set up "a cancer research fund along lines that will be approved by you," and expressed gratitude for her efforts in getting the donation.

Eric Johnston became chairman of the Society's new governing board, which was later renamed the Executive Committee. This high-powered group included James Adams, president of Standard Brands, Inc.; Elmer Bobst, president of Hoffmann-LaRoche, Inc., Emerson Foote, president of Foote, Cone & Belding (successors to Albert Lasker's Lord & Thomas); Morgan Brainard, president of Aetna Life Insurance Company; Thomas Braniff, president of Braniff Airlines; Lewis Douglas, president of Mutual Life Insurance Company; and Albert Lasker. Most active were Bobst, Adams, the Laskers, and Foote; the latter was vice-chairman. This committee was given responsibility for the funds and administration of the Society. A new professional committee to govern medical and scientific policies was also created.

In 1944 the Executive Committee reorganized the Society so that the board of directors would always be equally divided between laymen and medical/scientific professionals.

And Emerson Foote provided it with a new name: the American Cancer Society, Inc. "As an advertising man, it seemed to me that the American Society for the Control of Cancer was too long and awkward, hard to remember," Mr. Foote recalled recently. "American Cancer Society was simple and more direct. There was quite a bit of resistance to the change. Some doctors thought it implied that the Society was in favor of cancer, which was rather silly. Eventually it was accepted."

The newly named ACS faced an immediate problem: There was little money for support materials for the upcoming 1945 campaign. In August 1944 Mrs. Lasker was lunching with Emerson Foote to discuss this problem when she spotted an old friend in the restaurant—Lois Mattox Miller, medical editor of *Reader's Digest* magazine.

They briefed Mrs. Miller about the lack of cancer research, and the fact that a large percentage of Americans would die of cancer. With Foote's help, Mrs. Miller wrote a short piece for the October 1949 issue of the magazine. Headlined "Some Facts of Life-and-Death Interest to You," it began "Roughly, one out of six of you who read this will die of cancer," Emerson Foote recalled almost verbatim forty years later. Mrs. Miller had asked her editor in chief, DeWitt Wallace, for permission to add one line soliciting funds for the Society. The *Digest* had not previously opened its editorial pages to purposes, but Mr. Wallace agreed to make an exception because of the urgency of the need.

Foote recalls that the piece brought in $84,000 for the Society. Even Albert Lasker was impressed. According to Donald E. Shaughnessy, an early Society historian, this and two other short essays by Mrs. Miller in the *Digest* produced a total of $120,000.

Lee Casey unexpectedly resigned in the midst of the 1945 fund-raising campaign, apparently unused to coping with the mass of detail. Mrs. Lasker offered to hire and pay professional fund-raisers if 25 percent of all funds raised were earmarked for research. Her offer was accepted, and this has been the minimum percentage of ACS funds spent on research ever since. In subsequent campaigns the Society raised its own money.

The first fund-raising campaign of the American Cancer Society in 1945 brought in more than $4 million, of which a quarter—$1 million—was earmarked for research. At the time, the federal government was spending only $750,000 on cancer research, and in the entire country cancer research was receiving only about $1.5 million per year.

Although the Society now had money to spend on research, it had no program or machinery to administer. Its leaders asked the National Research Council to appoint a committee to take this responsibility.

The council created a fourteen-member Committee on Growth; the name was selected because it was felt that the problem of cancer was so broad and so basic that research into the disease would mean delving into the most fundamental aspects of life. There were four subsections: chemistry, biology, physics, and clinical investigations; later a section on chemotherapy was added. Appointed to the committee, made up of the country's leading cancer clinicians and scientists, were four members of the ACS board of directors: Drs. Little, Murphy, Morton, and Rhoads.

This led to a serious clash between the high-powered business executives on the Executive Committee and the physicians who had for so long controlled the Society. Adams, Bobst, and Lasker were particularly angered by the palpable conflict of interest: The four physicians were part of a group advising the Society about research projects, and were also members of the ACS board of directors who voted on these projects. The Executive Committee insisted that the doctors resign from the ACS board. There was the beginning of an ugly confrontation. The doctors were obdurate, the businessmen insistent. Finally James Adams approached Dr. Adair, who was trusted by both groups. Adair felt that the executives were right, but assured his four medical colleagues that their resignations would not be permitted to weaken the medical policies of ACS; that he would protect their interests. Then they wrote out their resignations.

Not only were there funds to stimulate research, the ACS also increased support for education, both professional and public, and for its program of service to the cancer patient— such as transportation of indigent patients and loans of hospital materials to be used at home.

The Society's leaders appointed a Committee on Reorganization in May 1945 to revise its bylaws. The committee recommended transferring all authority to the lay members by making them a majority on the board of directors, with responsibility for all activities of the Society via the Executive Committee. The doctors, however, refused to give over so much authority, although the new bylaws would still reserve direction of the professional programs to them. According to Donald Shaughnessy, they "threatened to bolt the Society en masse."

They made their point. The bylaws finally adopted on March 28, 1946, enlarged the board of directors to fifty-six, divided equally between scientific/medical and lay members. The powerful Executive Committee was expanded to nineteen, of which at least nine had to be laymen—thus giving doctors the deciding vote. The president, under the new bylaws, would always be a scientist or physician; the chairman of the board a layman.

A system of independent chartered and incorporated divisions of the Society was set up. In principle each would be statewide, but because of existing structures a few divisions represented metropolitan areas (such as New York City and Washington, D.C.). Thus, by the end of 1946, there were fifty-nine divisions in forty-eight states and the District of Columbia. (There are currently fifty-eight divisions in fifty states.) Divisions were put in charge of public and professional education, service, and fund-raising activities within their areas.

For local operations the Society was generally organized

by county-wide groups known as units. About a half-million volunteers worked in the units. There are today 3,242 ACS units with about 2,500,000 volunteers.

The Women's Field Army, headed by Mrs. Lucy Milligan since 1943, when Mrs. Illig resigned, maintained its integrity within the reorganized ACS, but its functions were gradually absorbed by the restructured organization. It became part of the Medical and Scientific Division, and its fund-raising, which had been the mainstay of the organization until 1944, receded in importance. In 1951 the office of national commander of the Field Army was discontinued; a corporate vice-presidency was created in its place, and it was stipulated that the office be held only by a woman. Many of the Field Army became Society volunteers; volunteer recruitment and training were given to the Department of Field Relations in the Society. In a farewell to the army, Dr. Little said, "It has made a breach in the wall of fear and ignorance concerning cancer which surrounded the American people."

VII

The New Executive Vice-President

One morning in the late 1940s, Mrs. Madelyn Worthing walked into the Utah State National Bank, in Salt Lake City, to see Lane Adams, a young assistant cashier. Her mission: to persuade him to become the state chairman of the American Cancer Society's Cancer Crusade.

Why Adams? "Darned if I know," Mr. Adams said recently. "I was a banker, and bankers are supposed to be community-minded. I was a joiner, headed the Red Cross drive, active on the zoo board and the Junior Chamber of Commerce, the local hospital board. I said to Mrs. Worthing, 'I think I've got so many obligations, I'm not sure I can take on any more.' She indicated that 'we' were aware of what I was doing, and thought I could handle one more thing.

"I asked for time to think it over, consulted with some of my friends. Mrs. Worthing's husband was an important depositor. And she asked several of her friends in the Cancer Society to apply pressure—I had many calls saying, 'I hope you'll give this favorable consideration.' I accepted."

At that time the ACS had regional representatives on its board of directors. That is, there were seven regions, each with its own board of directors, executive committee, and assembly. The assemblies met to elect a director to represent the region on the national board. Mr. Adams remained active in the Utah Division, rising to its presidency. Over the next ten years, he attended several ACS regional meetings, and

41

was elected to the national board. "After a couple of years, the board discovered I was a banker," he says, "and one day I became the national treasurer."

At the same time, the executive director of the Society, the late Mefford R. Runyon, a former CBS executive, had indicated his desire to take early retirement. A committee of three board members was elected to search for his successor: Governor Walter Kohler of Wisconsin; Dr. Eugene Pendergrass, director of the Department of Radiology at the University of Pennsylvania in Philadelphia; and Lane Adams. A letter was set to all division presidents asking for suggestions for a replacement for Mr. Runyon; and a professional executive recruiter canvassed foundations, universities, and government bureaus. Candidates were interviewed by the committee.

At one of their meetings in New York City, Governor Kohler asked permission to read a letter. It was from the president of the Utah Division of the ACS, Walter Jones, who suggested that Lane Adams be considered. "Without my advice or consent or knowledge," Mr. Adams said. "I told the governor, 'Well, that's ridiculous. Let's file it and move on to the next.' "

But after the meeting Kohler spoke seriously to him about the needs of the Cancer Society, and the opportunities of the position. Adams thought the possibility of his taking it was extremely remote, but promised to discuss it with his wife. Elaine Adams was unexpectedly positive about the job, although it meant taking two children out of school and moving to New York. Adams spoke to two Utah State Bank officers. Both attempted to discourage him. The bank's president urged him not to leave, pointing out that Adams was his logical successor.

One of the reasons Lane Adams considered the ACS job was that Mary Lasker, for whom he had great respect, insisted he take it. Since she and Elmer Bobst, James Adams, and Emerson Foote had reorganized the Society, it had grown enormously—its annual budget now surpassed $30 million. But growth had stretched the Society's staff and volunteer committee structure almost beyond their capacity to allocate funds and supervise programs. It was time to rebuild the staff.

As volunteer director and treasurer, Adams knew all this, but he felt a certain responsibility to deal with it. Besides, "I thought the job would only take about three years, long enough to reorganize the structure." After that, he could return to Utah and resume his banking career. With some misgivings, he accepted the ACS post of executive vice-president in 1959.

The Adamses left their daughter in school in Salt Lake City and came to New York with their son in September. "I was very disillusioned with what I found," Lane Adams recalls. "I wondered if I'd made a mistake. There was rivalry, bickering, jealousy, and animosity—a very uncharitable attitude of divisions toward the national office, of big cities toward divisions. The division executives were having a meeting in Estes Park, Colorado, just on the eve of my departure for New York. They asked me to attend; part of their agenda was to organize what you might call a 'union of executives,' indicative of the kind of attitude that was widespread throughout the Society. Who was this Adams guy? They were persuaded to postpone any action until they had a chance to appraise me, to see what made me tick."

At the national office, the chief medical officer, Dr. Harold S. Diehl, was in poor health; and the head of research, Dr. Harry Weaver, was about to leave. "It was not a very strong management team that I inherited," Mr. Adams recalls. "We had to attract and keep professionals. We needed a better salary structure, pension plan, and other things to compete for and hold talent. We had to make the ACS an attractive career."

He traveled a good deal to divisions to explain his agenda. And there were countless meetings with division executives to discuss management problems and relationships between divisions and the national office. It required enormous patience and diplomacy to knit them into a tighter national entity, to create a more efficient organization.

And there were other, even more pressing problems.

PART TWO

Controversies

VIII

The Smoking Gun

In 1937, while a graduate student at Johns Hopkins University, E. Cuyler Hammond studied under Professor Raymond Pearl, the father of biostatistics in the United States. Dr. Pearl had analyzed U.S. death rates with the help of Hammond and other students and found them rising. Since U.S. life expectancy was relatively low at the time—about sixty-two years—the most probable cause of this increase would have been cardiovascular disease, Dr. Hammond recalls. Cancer, which usually takes many years to develop, was unlikely to account for the rise.

Then Professor Pearl compared the death rates of smokers and nonsmokers of all forms of tobacco, and found, surprisingly, that heavy smokers had a life expectancy significantly shorter than that of nonsmokers. He published this information in an article in *Science* under the title "Tobacco Smoking and Longevity."

His paper was much criticized, and in fact a typical editorial in a leading American medical journal at the time stated that "extensive scientific studies have proved that smoking in moderation by those for whom tobacco is not especially contraindicated does not appreciably shorten life." This mirrored the prevailing medical opinion, and that of many scientists as well. However others had noted ominous connections between smoking and cancer. As early as 1859, a French physician, Bouisson, had done a retrospective study of sixty-eight cases of cancer of the oral cavity, and found that sixty-six had been tobacco smokers, the other two, tobacco

47

chewers. And in 1927 a British doctor, F. E. Tylecote, had reported that in almost every case of lung cancer he had seen or known about, the patient had been a heavy smoker of cigarettes. The Scandinavian countries had also noted an increase in lung cancer. In fact, as early as 1929, the Nordic Congress of Pathologists had reported a disquieting rise in lung-cancer deaths in Finland. But these European observations had gone largely unnoticed in the United States. At the time, European experience was not considered pertinent to America.

Chest surgeons were the first in the country to detect a phenomenal increase in lung cancer. One, Dr. Alton Ochsner of New Orleans, was to have a particularly powerful effect in linking smoking with this trend in the United States.

When Dr. Ochsner was a medical student at Washington University in St. Louis in 1919, his pathology professor had invited the class to witness an autopsy of a man who had died of lung cnacer. This was an unusual event, the professor, Dr. George Dock, had explained; they might never see another case of this extremely rare disease in a lifetime of medical practice.

"Seventeen years elapsed before I saw another case of lung cancer," Dr. Ochsner recalled later. It was 1936 and he was then professor of surgery at Tulane University in New Orleans. Two cases of an unusual cancer in seventeen years weren't startling, "but eight other cases were seen in a period of six months, which was extremely unusual. . . . All of the patients were men, they all smoked cigarettes heavily and had begun smoking in the first World War." Based on this personal observation, Dr. Ochsner deduced that a possible carcinogenic agent in tobacco smoke might have produced these cancers in about twenty years. He admitted that the evidence was "nebulous," but smoking cigarettes seemed the most likely cause.

Dr. Ochsner, who later became president of the American Cancer Society, told the International Cancer Congress in

1939: "It's our conviction that the increase in the incidence of pulmonary carcinoma is due largely to the increase in smoking, particularly cigarette smoking, which is universally associated with inhalation."

Such clinical observations continued to accumulate in the United States, England, and Scandinavia. They spurred the American Cancer Society to fund a "case-control" study of lung cancer and smoking in the late 1940s, at the Washington School of Medicine in St. Louis, Missouri. In this study, a group of lung-cancer patients was contrasted with a somewhat larger group of hospital patients without lung cancer, and their smoking histories were compared. The study director was Dr. Evarts A. Graham, the first surgeon to cure a case of human lung cancer by the daring operation of removing an entire lung. His associate was a medical student, now Dr. Ernst L. Wynder, head of the American Health Foundation.

Graham and Wynder studied 684 lung-cancer patients, almost all men, and 780 patients in hospitals with other diseases. They found that 94 percent of the people with lung cancers were cigarette smokers, 4 percent were pipe smokers, and 3.5 percent were cigar smokers. Only 2 percent were nonsmokers or smoked almost not at all. Among the non-lung-cancer patients, more than 14 percent were nonsmokers, and the number of heavy smokers was only half as great as among the people with lung cancer.

The authors' conclusion: "Extensive and prolonged use of tobacco, especially cigarettes, seems to be an important factor in the inducement of bronchogenic carcinoma."

Meanwhile, Cuyler Hammond had gone on to win his Sci.D. and to study biostatistical problems for a government agency. In 1947 he was hired by the American Cancer Society as director of statistical research and controls. His job was to assess the effectiveness of the Society's programs and to study statistical patterns of cancer mortality and morbidity.

Dr. Hammond had never forgotten his work with Raymond Pearl, and had followed the professional literature on trends in mortality. When analyzing death rates from cancer, he found that for nearly all forms of the disease the rates were flat or dropping, except for lung cancer. Mortality rates from these tumors were "rising at an alarming rate," he said not long ago. "There were three or four possible explanations. Best guess was something that got into the lungs. It might have been coal soot, or tar from roads: both substances had been shown to contain benzo-a-pyrenes, powerful carcinogens. Coal and fuel oil were being widely burned, and more and more people were driving on tarred road. The only other pertinent thing that was going up, that had been going up dramatically, was smoking cigarettes."

Hammond did a comparative study of these possibilities, and included the variation between urban and rural death rates. This eliminated coal soot—less coal was being burned—but the other three possibilities remained: oil, tar, and cigarettes, as well as a perhaps unknown cause of the higher urban death rate.

In order to evaluate the effects of smoking, Hammond wanted to do a "prospective" study—following people into the future—a relatively new concept in the late 1940s. He calculated that a study of this type would have to follow at least 100,000 white males, ages fifty to sixty-nine—the group at highest risk for lung cancer—both smokers and nonsmokers, for about four years to achieve statistically significant results.

There were no experts on prospective studies. No one had ever attempted to prospectively study a hundred thousand people, nor to follow them for several years. Hammond's friends told him that this was an impossible task and advised him not to try it. Scientists connected with the ACS were dubious. So were doctors on the ACS board. They felt that the results of such a study would be unreliable and might damage the Society's reputation.

However, Dr. Charles S. Cameron, the medical director, was a proponent. Dr. Cameron recalls being taken to lunch at

"21" by Elmer Bobst, president of Hoffmann-LaRoche and a prominent ACS board member, with an executive of the Reynolds Tobacco Company. Mr. Bobst, too, was concerned about the ACS's reputation, and the tobacco executive tried to convince Cameron that a young organization ought not to meddle in so complicated a subject, using a questionable method of research. But Cameron was unmoved, and convinced Bobst that the ACS project was sound. This was essential, for the board would have to vote money to underwrite it.

"I also got strong support from the ACS publicity people, headed by Clifton Read," Dr. Hammond recalls, "and the organization people. On the board, it was Jim Adams [of Lazard Frères] and Elmer Bobst who were most enthusiastic."

Hammond asked the Gallup and Roper polling organizations how much it would cost to interview a hundred thousand subjects. They estimated $50 per subject—an astronomical $5 million, which amounted to more than one-third of the total annual income of the ACS at the time. And neither organization was certain that it could trace a hundred thousand people for four years. It had never been done.

Dr. Hammond's wife then suggested using ACS volunteers as fieldworkers. At that time, Dr. Hammond recalls, the typical volunteer was a woman who had ended her professional career to get married. Many had been schoolteachers or well educated in other fields. "They were very intelligent women," Hammond says. "I also knew how little training most professional interviewers were given. So we decided to try to do our study with volunteers."

Dr. Hammond visited ten cities—among them Baltimore, Nashville, Denver, Chicago—and recruited about 200 volunteers for a trial run: They handed out 2,000 questionnaires and turned them in, all properly filled out. "Then we knew it could be done," Hammond says. He and his associate, Dr. Daniel Horn, with a young assistant statistician,

Lawrence Garfinkel, designed and tested a questionnaire for their study. Then they recruited 22,000 American Cancer Society volunteers in 394 counties in nine states: California, Illinois, Iowa, Michigan, Minnesota, New Jersey, New York, Pennsylvania, and Wisconsin. Each volunteer was asked to give the questionnaire to ten white males, between fifty and sixty-nine years old, whom she knew well and would be able to find each year.

"In 1950, when Hammond and Horn's study was first planned, few persons had much experience of applying epidemiological methods to the study of noninfectious diseases, and the large-scale cohort study, which is now so standard, was still in its infancy," wrote Sir Richard Doll in 1984. Dr. Doll, regius professor emeritus of medicine at the University of Oxford, is known as one of the top two or three cancer eidemiologists in the world.

The crucial factors, Doll noted, were "an ability to collect unbiased information about a sample of individuals with varying personal characteristics that was large enough for there to be a reasonable chance of detecting material differences in disease incidence between different subgroups within a period short enough for the results to be still of interest . . . and an ability to keep in touch with the individuals to record accurately [their] morbidity and mortality.

"Hammond and Horn had the imagination to see that both objectives could be achieved by enlisting the support of active members of the American Cancer Society. . . . They also had the confidence to feel able to handle the mass of data that would be accumulated . . . and extract the most crucial information without the sophisticated computer systems that now make such tasks relatively easy."

The volunteers came close to reaching their goal of ten questionnaires each—that would have been 220,000 questionnaires, more than twice Hammond's original estimate. Actually, they did turn in more than 204,000 questionnaires between January 1 and May 31, 1952. After winnowing by

Hammond and colleagues, 189,854 were found useful. Each year thereafter, starting November 1, 1952, and on the same date through 1955, the volunteers were asked to check the list of persons they had enrolled and report whether subjects were alive or dead. If dead, Hammond and Horn wrote to the health department in the state where the death occurred for a copy of the death certificate, which showed the cause of death. These were willingly supplied without charge because health authorities were interested in the results of this unique survey.

Analyzing the first two years of follow-up, which were phenomenally close to perfection—above 99 percent of subjects were traced—some amazing connections between cigarette smoking and major killing diseases began to emerge. So clear, in fact, were these connections that Dr. Hammond, who had been a three-pack-a-day cigarette smoker, Dr. Horn, who also smoked cigarettes, and Lawrence Garfinkel all gave up cigarettes. More important, Hammond felt compelled to inform medical professionals of the study's preliminary findings.

He did this on June 21, 1954, at the American Medical Association's convention in San Francisco. A two-pack-a-day smoker, he told the doctors, had a risk of lung cancer twenty-five times (2,500 percent) as great as that of a nonsmoker, as well as considerably increased risk of oral cancers. The other important finding was that cigarette smokers had twice as many coronary heart attacks as nonsmokers.

The paper created shock waves worldwide and was front-page news from New York to Tokyo. The headline on page one of the *New York Times* on Tuesday, June 22, 1954, beneath a top-of-page, three-column photograph of Drs. Hammond and Horn, read: CIGARETTES FOUND TO RAISE DEATH RATE IN MEN 50 TO 70. The story, by Lawrence E. Davies, ran about two full columns and said in part:

> Cigarette smokers from 50 to 70 years of age have a death
> rate from all causes as much as 75 percent higher than that of

nonsmokers, the American Cancer Society reported today. . . .

Deaths among smokers . . . were mainly from cancer and heart attack, the study showed. . . .

The American Cancer Society had started at least a five year study, and had not expected to make a public finding before next year. Dr. E. Cuyler Hammond . . . said, however, "We found cigarette smokers had so much higher death rates that we didn't think we should withhold the information another year."

The *New York Times* handles news conservatively. Other papers were more sensational. The result was that many people stopped smoking cigarettes, at least temporarily, and cigarette sales dropped. It was the beginning of what the tobacco industry calls the "health scare." The companies' immediate reaction was to try to offer a "safer" product. They began to add filters to cigarettes. In 1954, filter-tipped cigarettes made up only about 5 percent of sales; in the 1980s, 95 percent of U.S. cigarettes were filter-tipped.

Fieldwork for the Hammond-Horn study was finished by the end of October 1955. The material for a forty-four-month follow-up of a final total of 187,783 men was assembled on punch cards. Only 1.1 percent had been lost to follow-up. The total experience included 667,753 man years. In the interim, 11,870 of the subjects had died, and death certificates were obtained for all. The study was unprecedented in size, scope, and completeness—a success far greater than the Hammond-Horn team had anticipated in their most euphoric moments.

Sir Richard Doll reassessed the work in the *Journal of the American Medical Association* thirty years later, in June 1984. Calling it a "remarkable enterprise," Dr. Doll wrote:

Hammond and Horn's study broke new ground in two ways. First, it showed that it was possible to elicit useful information about personal habits from as many as 200,000 persons, follow them up for several years, and obtain information about their causes of death. Second, it showed that smoking was associated with a much wider variety of ills than had been previously suspected, that the association was, in nearly all cases, much closer for smoking cigarettes than for smoking tobacco in other forms, and that among regular cigarette smokers, smoking might be responsible for up to 40% of their total mortality.

The Hammond-Horn study was published in two parts in the *Journal of the American Medical Association* in March 1958. In an unusual tribute, the *Journal* republished part two as a "Landmark article" in June 1984, and the American Medical association voted a special commendation to the authors.

IX

The Gun Goes Off

Between 1954, when the preliminary results of the Hammond-Horn study were first announced (in June) and then published (August) in the *Journal of the American Medical Association*, and 1958, when the completed study was finally published, a great debate began within the American Cancer Society. Until then the Society had been primarily a medium for funneling medical information from physicians and scientific sources to the public and the medical profession. It had begun creating new information when it started funding scientific investigations in 1945. But these too, were independent of the Society. Now, for the first time, it had turned out an original and groundbreaking piece of research by its own volunteers and staff. More important, the findings had implications for the public far greater and more disturbing than any single research project until that time.

The question was whether the Society, on the basis of its own discoveries, should become more than a passive conduit for information; whether, in fact, it should not become an activist organization.

A critical observer of U.S. philanthropies, Richard Carter, wrote:

> When it finally discovered that smoking was statistically associated with ill health, especially lung cancer, the society found itself in a painful position. The statistics invited it to tangle with one of the country's most affluent industries, and inform millions of Americans that one of their favorite pastimes had suicidal aspects. No voluntary health agency had ever engaged

56

in such controversy. The effect on fund raising promised to be negative. The effect on the medical profession was hardly to be anticipated with relish: numerous doctors were already annoyed at the society because patients were lately asking for "cancer examinations" (as if doctors needed instruction from patients), and now doctors were to be embarrassed by their own habitual smoking.

To exhort the nation to seek medical attention was one thing. To become a public spoilsport and common scold was quite another. The society leadership was tempted to be conservative: nobody had yet *proved* that tobacco smoke caused lung cancer. Perhaps the society should wait for actual proof or soft-pedal the statistical association demonstrated in the survey. Or forget the whole unappetizing project.

The ACS created an ad hoc committee on tobacco and cancer, and in October 1954 the committee adopted a resolution stating that: "available evidence indicates an association between smoking, particularly cigarette smoking, and lung cancer and to a lesser degree other forms of cancer." Committee resolutions, however, are not official positions of the Society unless they are adopted by the national board of directors. And there were grave doubts as to whether this would take place.

The ACS had become, of course, a national organization. It had volunteers and divisions and units in every state—including the tobacco states. Some of its adherents were tobacco farmers, or worked for the large tobacco companies. Others were in the wholesale or retail tobacco trade. For these people, even being connected with an organization that sponsored the Hammond-Horn study created conflicts that involved their livelihood. But starting an active antismoking program was much more serious. There were resignations and recriminations.

Too, ACS medical and scientific policy has always been dominated by physicians and researchers who are, by the nature of their training and professional responsibilities, conservative. In addition, as Mr. Carter noted, many were themselves heavy smokers. The Hammond-Horn study had produced shocking information, but it was the first study of its kind. Were its conclusions sufficiently reliable to support basic ACS policy changes? There was then scanty biomedical proof that cigarette smoke caused cancer in animals or in humans. The instinct of the organization's medical/scientific leaders was to move slowly, to do more studies, to be sure of their ground.

Lane Adams, volunteer and treasurer of the ACS in the 1950s, recalls that there was "division within the board, whether we should be taking the kind of definitive action we did in going on record as saying that cigarette smoking is the cause of lung cancer. That really shook up the establishment.

The board chairman, James Adams, who was also the investment counsel of the Lasker family, was a staunch ally of Cuyler Hammond. And Dr. Howard C. Taylor, Jr., son of one of the Society's founders, and later, like his father, president of the ACS, was also out in front on this issue: "We had a battle on the board of directors," he recalled nearly twenty years later. "The laymen opposed [a resolution saying that tobacco was a significant cause of lung cancer]." But, of course, James Adams and Bobst were laymen and at the same time proponents of a strong anticigarette statement. Besides, the genie was already out of the bottle. And the Society has always had a tradition of freedom of speech for its staff. No one had considered blocking Hammond from publicizing his results or publishing his study; no one had attempted to influence him to suppress or change his conclusions. Dr. Charles S. Cameron, ACS medical and scientific director and himself a smoker, did not share Hammond's convictions, but Dr. Hammond recalls that Cameron was nevertheless very supportive.

Hammond pushed hard for action, standing up at ACS committee and board meetings to say that "these lives are on my conscience."

Perhaps the strongest proponent of an unequivocal statement on smoking and health was Dr. Alton Ochsner. Lane
Adams, the executive vice-president of ACS, from 1959 to
1985, recalls that Dr. Ochsner, who was ACS president in
1958, listened to the debate and then told a story. It was
about a Russian count who suspected his wife of infidelity. In
order to verify, or allay, his suspicions, the count pretended to
leave on a journey, but actually he returned stealthily and
took up a position from where he could observe through field
glasses what went on in his house. Hardly had he stationed
himself when a carriage drove up and a handsome young man
got out and went into the count's house. The countess
greeted him and took his coat and hat. Soon the lights went
on in an upstairs bedroom. Through the window, the count
could see the visitor with his wife. The man removed his
outer garments, and then the lights went out and he could
could see no more. "Ah," he said, "if I could only be sure. As
it is, I can only doubt."

Dr. Ochsner, who was a wonderful raconteur, got the
board's full attention with his story and had them all laughing
at the punch line. "Doubt, doubt, doubt," he said, and called
for a vote on the tobacco issue. The board voted overwhelm-
ingly for a strong statement.

From then on, the tobacco companies perceived the
American Cancer Society as the enemy. It is no exaggeration
to use the David/Goliath analogy. The ACS had several
powerful people on its board, but had never been supported
by industry in general. The tobacco companies represented a
$6,182,000,000 industry with enormous political influence.
Tobacco is a cash crop in sixteen states and dominates the
economies of at least two—North Carolina and Kentucky.
Tobacco-supported congressmen were generally reelected
time after time, and therefore had seniority on key committees. They gave the cigarette companies enormous political
clout. Tobacco influence extended to all communications
media because of the huge collective advertising budgets of

the cigarette companies. They were also beginning to diversify, to buy up other industries, whose economic power pyramided that of tobacco.

In short, the Society had taken on a formidable opponent with resources and influence far greater than anything it could muster. It had one powerful resource: the link between smoking and ill health, which was growing stronger every day.

The Society tried to persuade the surgeon general of the U.S. Public Health Service to take a stand on smoking, and in 1957 the then surgeon general, Dr. Leroy Burney, did prepare such a statement. However, he was prevented from publishing it for two years by bureaucratic red tape, and when he did finally release a watered-down version in an article in the *Journal of the American Medical Association* in 1959, it was generally ignored.

Stronger ammunition was needed, and Cuyler Hammond decided to seek it. With Lawrence Garfinkel, he began constructing the largest prospective epidemiological study the world had ever seen. Called the Cancer Prevention Study (CPS), it would, like the smoking study, depend on the devotion and dedication of ACS volunteers as fieldworkers. It was planned to begin with a questionnaire that elicited 300 bits of information to be supplied by at least 1 million Americans over age thirty. Separate forms for men and women covered everything from age, occupation, and marital status to such intimate details as whether they had blood in the urine, diarrhea, or unusual vaginal discharge. Subjects would then be followed by the volunteer researchers for at least six years, and for those who died, death certificates would be sought.

There were serious doubts as to whether many people would provide such personal information. However, when the questionnaire was tested in five cities by ACS volunteers, and the purpose of the survey was explained, all questions were answered. The information would of course be confidential; the forms were mailed directly to ACS headquarters by the subjects in coded brown envelopes supplied by the fieldworkers.

Meanwhile, the ACS board of directors voted to initiate a powerful antismoking campaign among grade- and high-school students. First priority were those who had not yet become habitual smokers. Based on a study of 22,000 high-school students in Portland, Oregon, programs were aimed at teaching teachers via workshops and getting materials into various school courses. Throughout the country there were film showings with physician speakers, student discussions, science experiments, antismoking assembly programs. There were also local and regional youth conferences and youth press conferences that students helped to plan and run.

In 1960 the Society was ready to state: "Beyond a reasonable doubt cigarette smoking is the major cause of the unprecedented increase in lung cancer." Lung-cancer mortality in the United States was then 36,420. The ACS estimated that by 1972 the number of lung-cancer deaths would have nearly doubled.

The Cancer Prevention study had begun in 1959, with the recruitment of 68,000 ACS volunteer researchers in twenty-nine states. They persuaded 1,051,443 men and women to fill out questionnaires and successfully followed 98.4 percent of them for six years. The nearly perfect follow-up of so many people for so many years was a phenomenal achievement. "Even hospitals have difficulty tracing cancer patients for five years." Dr. Hammond noted, "and commercial organizations would not undertake to follow the large number of subjects enrolled in the ACS study."

One volunteer wrote seventeen letters to track down a single subject, a Catholic nun registered in the Midwest who had moved to Guatemala. One male subject told a fieldworker that he didn't know where his wife was: "She's gone off with another man." Mobile-home dwellers were particularly hard to trace. And perhaps the most difficult of all was a man who was somewhere in Canada but left no clue to his whereabouts.

The researcher was relieved to learn that this subject was also wanted by the Royal Canadian Northwest Mounted Police.

During the six years of follow-up, 75,847 deaths were reported among subjects, and death certificates were obtained for 75,528, (99.6 percent). Every other year during the study, volunteers distributed short supplementary questionnaires requesting more information on illnesses, hospitalization, and other matters. More than 95 percent of subjects still alive in 1965 answered and returned these questionnaires. Altogether, CPS produced more than 450 million pieces of information, which are stored on thirty-five rolls of magnetic computer tape. And the study was reactivated in 1971–72, six years after the last follow-up—that is, thirteen years after CPS began—to gain more cancer statistics, because it takes most cancers a great many years to develop.

Volunteers and only volunteers were able to do this huge, long-term prospective population study with a degree of completeness and accuracy close to perfection. There was the question of economy. Estimates from professional polling organizations, multiplied by the follow-ups, would have placed the total price of fieldwork at about $300 million for the first six years of CPS, and at least as much for the later follow-up. Not even the federal government had that kind of budget for surveys of this type.

Nearly 100 separate studies have been mined from the mass of data produced by this huge investigation. Among them were a number that provided further proof of the relationship between cigarette smoking and cancer and other diseases and pathological conditions.

One key probe using CPS data answered the often-asked question as to whether the association between cigarette smoking and higher death rates might have resulted from an accidental relationship between smoking and some other factor that influences death rates. This study is based on a "matched-pair analysis," wherein 36,975 pairs of male smokers and nonsmokers were extracted from the more than

420,000 male subjects in the CPS. These pairs were matched by computer in nineteen ways, except in smoking habits: They were alike in race, height, nativity, residence, occupation, education, marital status, consumption of alcohol, and eleven other criteria. After three years of follow-up of these pairs, the following was noted:

- Twice as many of the smokers had died of all causes—1,385 deaths among the smokers, as against 662 deaths of nonsmokers.
- There were 110 lung-cancer deaths among the smokers, as against only 12 lung-cancer deaths among the nonsmokers.
- More than twice as many smokers had died of coronary heart disease—654, as against 304 coronary deaths among the nonsmokers.

The study also revealed other striking differences in death rates between men alike in almost every way except for smoking. The smokers died more frequently from emphysema and cancers of the mouth, pharynx, larynx, esophagus, pancreas, and bladder.

X

The Government Joins the Battle

On June 1, 1961, Dr. John W. Cline, president of the American Cancer Society; Dr. Oglesby Paul, president of the American Heart Association; Miss Marion W. Sheahan, R.N., president of the American Public Health Association; and Mr. Herbert C. DeYoung, president of the National Tuberculosis Association (now the American Lung Asssociation) wrote a joint letter to President John F. Kennedy outlining some of the health dangers of cigarette smoking and pointing out that the resulting damage would be huge in terms of loss of life and cost in economic productivity "unless appropriate measures are taken.

"The voluntary agencies have acted and used their resources to uncover, define and explain the health risks of cigarette smoking," the letter continued. "But the widespread implications of the tobacco problem extend far beyond the capabilities of voluntary agencies. . . . [W]e respectfully request that you appoint a commission to consider it."

A little over a month later, on July 7, 1961, Luther K. Terry, M.D., surgeon general of the U.S. Public Health Service, announced that he was appointing a medical and scientific committee to undertake a comprehensive review of all data on smoking and health.

The committee was composed of 10 expert physicians and scientists, representing all disciplines related to the problem. These men were picked with the approval of both the tobacco industry and public-health groups. They were

Stanhope Bayne-Jones, M.D., Ph.D., Yale and Cornell Universities. Field: Nature and Causation of Disease in Human Populations.

Walter J. Burdette, M.D., Ph.D., University of Utah. Fields: Surgery, Genetics.

William G. Cochran, M.A., Harvard University. Field: Biological Statistics.

Emmanuel Farber, M.D., Ph.D., University of Pittsburgh. Field: Pathology.

Louis F. Feiser, Ph.D., Harvard University. Field: Chemistry of Carcinogenic Hydrocarbons.

Jacob Furth, M.D., Columbia University. Field: Cancer Biology.

John H. Hickam, M.D., University of Indiana. Fields: Internal Medicine, Physiology and Cardiopulmonary Disease, Preventive Medicine.

Charles LeMaistre, M.D., University of Texas. Fields: Internal Medicine, Pulmonary Diseases, Preventive Medicine.

Leonard M. Schuman, M.D., University of Minnesota. Field: Epidemiology.

Maurice H. Seevers, M.D., Ph.D., University of Michigan. Field: Pharmacology of Anesthesia and Habit-Forming Drugs.

Under Luther Terry, the committee studied 1,100 research reports on smoking and health, and a summary of 6,000 other such studies. The committee also called on 175 experts for help in special areas. Among them, Cuyler Hammond. At this point the CPS had had two annual follow-ups; Hammond and Garfinkel prepared an interim analysis of the data to that time. This confirmed in many ways the relationship between cigarette smoking and disease found in the

Hammond-Horn study. It had great impact on the committee's final 367-page report on smoking and health, issued on January 11, 1964, which has since been known as the "Surgeon General's Report."

There were two major conclusions:

1. "Cigarette smoking is a health hazard of sufficient importance in the United States to warrant remedial action" and
2. "Cigarette smoking is causally related to lung cancer in men; the magnitude of the effect of cigarette smoking far outweighs other factors. The data for women, although less extensive, point in the same direction."

The report also stated that smoking was "one of the most important causes of chronic bronchitis in the United States and increases the risk of dying from chronic bronchitis and emphysema," and pointed out that "male cigarette smokers have a higher death rate from coronary artery disease than nonsmokers."

The "Surgeon General's Report" had a shock value similar to that of the first atomic bomb: The reverberations will apparently never cease. Dr. Terry said later that the evening after the report was released "we saw camera coverage on every televsion network and station and the next morning we found front-page coverage in every newspaper in the country. Later we saw that this coverage had reached across the world."

The committee was "jubilant . . . we thought maybe we had 'conquered' cigarette smoking." But the habit was more tenacious than they imagined. Although there was a precipitous drop in cigarette sales for a few days, soon they were up again.

The report did, however, add a new dimension to the controversy: It was the first time that the U.S. government had taken a policy stance against smoking in an official document. The Public Health Service established a National Clearinghouse on Smoking and Health in 1965; under Dr. Daniel Horn, formerly of the ACS, it sponsored behavioral research on smoking and quitting, and provided educational information and scientific reports of research in the field from all over the world. Not the least of its efforts went to helping the surgeon general prepare comprehensive reports on smoking and health now required annually by Congress. In recent years many of the reports have delved in depth into separate pathologies. Cumulatively they have added to and strengthened the conclusions of the first "Surgeon General's Report." Some key findings:

- According to a recent assessment by the U.S. assistant secretary for health, Dr. Edward N. Brandt, Jr., **"Cigarette smoking is the major single cause of cancer in the United States.** Tobacco's contribution to *all* cancer deaths is estimated to be 30 percent," Tobacco-genic cancers include not only lung cancer but also cancers of the larynx, oral cavity, esophagus, bladder, kidney, pancreas, stomach, and even the uterine cervix.
- Smokers have significantly shorter life expectancy on average than nonsmokers—eight and three-tenths fewer years for a twenty-five-year-old two-pack-a-day smoker.

A recent report focused on cardiovascular disease, and stated for the first time in a government document that cigarette smoking "is *a major cause of coronary heart disease (CHD) in the United States for both men and women* [our italics]. . . . [It] should be considered the most important of the known modifiable risk factors for CHD. [Smoking is] estimated responsible for up to 30 percent of CHD deaths in the United States each year [i.e., about 170,000 fatal heart attacks annually]. "The report estimates "three million premature deaths from heart disease among Americans between 1965 and 1980," and goes on to say that, cigarette smoking "has a significant positive association with atherosclerosis [deposits of cholesterol in arteries]." There is evidence that cigarette smoke alters cholesterol levels and affects platelet function. Platelets are blood-clotting factors, and experimental data show that smoking causes them to stick together, making them more likely to form a clot. Blood clots are implicated in many heart attacks.

During these years of increasingly stronger government statements, the private agencies expanded their activities against smoking. A National Interagency Council on Smoking and Health was established by a number of national voluntary organizations with an interest in the field—most notably the ACS, the American Heart Association, and the American Lung Association. The ACS wrote to college presidents, questioning the propriety of cigarette advertising in college publications; the cigarette companies voluntarily relinquished such advertising in 1963. The Society also made films for general audiences and TV spots against smoking, and sponsored literally millions of meetings at which films were shown and speakers enlightened audiences about smoking and health.

In 1965, Congress passed the first law regulating the labeling of cigarettes (which are specifically exempted by law from regulation by the Food and Drug Administration) sold within the United States (but not for export): "Caution: Cigarette smoking may be hazardous to your health." These warnings have, by act of Congress, become increasingly more specific and now, following the lead of Sweden, include four different messages. But the same law—reflecting lobbying pressure from the cigarette industry—barred the Federal Trade Commission (FTC) from demanding warnings in cigarette advertising for four years. The FTC established a laboratory to analyze tar and nicotine content of U.S. cigarettes, but the information was kept secret until 1969. It is now published semiannually, along with, in more recent years, assays of carbon monoxide (CO) in the smoke of the various brands. European countries had begun doing this because of the link established between CO and cardiovascular disease.

There had been antismoking movements in various countries for many years—based largely on religious motivations. But after the Hammond-Horn study, more serious medical/scientific statements and investigations gave new direction and force to these enterprises.

For example, in 1962 the British Royal College of Physicians published its own report on smoking and health, which stated unequivocally that "cigarette smoking is a cause of lung cancer and bronchitis and probably contributes to the development of coronary heart disease."

In 1963 twenty-five leading Swedish scientists and physicians petitioned their government to act against smoking. One result: The Swedish government became the first to fund a specialized agency on smoking and health.

In 1964 the Norwegian Parliament voted *unanimously* for an active national campaign against smoking (the U.S. Congress has never made a similar statement).

In subsequent years the three Nordic governments— Norway, Sweden, Finland—and leading private institutions have taken a whole series of actions against smoking: banning most tobacco advertising, permitting no advertising for any product in which models smoke, forbidding smoking in many public places, making teaching about smoking and disease mandatory in all schools.

To illustrate how universal was the problem of smoking and health, and how it was dealt with by many countries, in 1967 the American Cancer Society helped to organize the first World Conference on Smoking and Health. Attending were 511 delegates from thirty-two countries and forty-two U.S. states—an impressive group that helped increase public awareness worldwide. International meetings of this type have since been held every four years: After the third conference, the Society began to publish and distribute worldwide, without charge, the first journal devoted to the social, economic, political, and organized-cessation aspects of smoking: *World Smoking and Health.*

In 1967 in the United States, John Bahnzaf, an activist law professor at Georgetown University in Washingotn, D.C., petitioned the Federal Communications Commission (FCC), which regulates all broadcasting over public channels, to apply the "fairness doctrine" to cigarette advertising. Briefly, this concept holds that if a radio or television station gives or sells time for a political message, it must provide time for the opposition. The FCC ruled that in the case of cigarette advertising, stations or networks would have to broadcast one antismoking spot at no charge for every four paid cigarette commercials. Between June 1967 and the end of 1971 the ACS distributed more than 2,200 prints of TV spots, and countless radio tapes. Other organizations also contributed messages. Altogether, the major TV networks telecast well over 5,000 such spots in prime time as a public service.

About 10 million more smokers quit during those four years than normally would have stopped smoking through attrition (usually because of dangerous symptoms or serious disease). However, this antismoking broadcast bonanza disappeared in 1971 when the FTC persuaded Congress to ban all cigarette advertising from radio and TV—(as had already been done in the Nordic countries and eight others, including Great Britain, Italy, Switzerland, and the Soviet Union).

All of these activities can be classified as societal or political. The tobacco interests were constantly critical: There was no direct, biomedical evidence that cigarette smoke could produce lung cancer in large animals, much less in human beings. In 1955 Cuyler Hammond and Lawrence Garfinkel teamed up with a well-known pathologist, Dr. Oscar Auerbach of the Veterans Administration, to try to fill this gap with a series of animal and human pathological studies.

The first such animal study in 1967 was of beagle dogs. These were divided into groups, smoking number of cigarettes equivalent to one to two packs a day by a 150-pound man, plus a nonsmoking control group. The experiments went on for 875 days, during which time a number of dogs died, none of them in the nonsmoking group. At the end of the experiments, two of eight nonsmoking dogs had lung tumors; four of ten dogs who smoked filter-tipped cigarettes had tumors; five of ten of a group of nonfilter-cigarette-smoking dogs who smoked only half as many cigarettes, and twelve of twelve in the full-quota nonfilter group, had tumors. Invasive tumors were found only in full-quota nonfilter-smoking dogs, and two of these were similar to the type of carcinomas most often seen in the lungs of human male smokers.

The same team did retrospective blind pathological studies of the lungs, larynxes, and arterioles (small blood vessels) of several thousand men who had died of a variety of causes. In these "blind" studies, the tissues were examined by pathologists who did not know the men's smoking histories until after they had noted the condition of the tissues. Then the tissue slides were matched with the smoking habits of the subjects. In all cases, smokers turned out to have a preponderance of thickened arteries, abnormal laryngeal cells, and lung pathologies. In the lung study, the relationship was clearly established as one of dose-response—the more the men smoked, and the longer they had smoked, the more evidence of tissue damage.

THE SMOKE SCENE

After cigarette advertising was barred from U.S. broadcasts, broadcasters were no longer required to give special air time to antismoking messages. And they have greatly reduced the number of such messages. At the same time, tobacco companies have managed to partially subvert the broadcast ban by taking large billboard spaces to advertise cigarettes near scoreboards in baseball and football stadiums, where TV cameras cannot avoid their messages; underwriting tennis tournaments and other sports events so that their brand names become part of the reporting of the event; and putting decals on racing cars and drivers' coveralls.

Most magazines and newspapers do not publish many articles or cover much news linking smoking with ill health. For these print media, cigarette advertising is often the difference between profit and loss. Tobacco advertising totals over $1.5 billion a year in the United States, which gives the tobacco companies great economic leverage over editorial policies. Even on the airwaves the tobacco companies have power; they are still able to advertise cigars and pipe tobacco. They have also diversified into dog food, aluminum foil, container shipping, packaged food, scotch whisky, beer, and a variety of other products that have substantial advertising budgets and can be advertised via radio and TV. Through these additional advertising budgets, the tobacco companies can also exert great influence in broadcasting.

To combat this prosmoking force, the American Cancer Society has attempted to educate the American people—with heavy concentration in grade and high schools—about smoking and health, and to help them quit. Perhaps its most visible and best-known campaign is the Great Annual American Smokeout. This began in a small town in Minnesota in 1973, and in 1976 the ACS made it a national event. It has grown each year since, creating so many newsworthy happenings that the media cannot ignore it. In 1984 a survey taken after the event projected that some 24 million Americans pledged to quit smoking for the day of November 21. The Smokeout now has counterparts in many foreign countries.

Massive changes have taken place in the American people's knowledge of the risks of smoking and the benefits of quitting, and in their behavior. Perhaps the best measure of the latter is that in a recent Gallup survey, only about twenty-nine percent of U.S. adults over age eighteen were found to be regular smokers: 31 percent of men, 28 percent of women. Contrast this with the fact that more than 50 percent of U.S. men smoked in 1963, and nearly one-third of adult U.S. women. If past trends had continued, there would be well over 80 million adult American smokers: as it is, there are about 50–55 million smokers. Even more impressive, for the past twelve years—after various rises and falls related to the Hammond/Horn study, the "Surgeon General's Report" and other events—the annual consumption of cigarettes by U.S. adults, eighteen and older, has moved steadily downward (as shown in the chart on page 74).

Cigarette sales in the United States have been dropping steadily. In 1981 they hit 636 billion; by 1982 they had declined to 632 billion; and in 1983 there was a sharp 8-percent drop to 584 billion. Anticipating these trends, the world's largest cigarette companies, mainly British and American, have in recent years been focusing their cigarette marketing, tobacco growing, and manufacturing efforts in the third world. Populations of third-world countries have begun to reflect this with a rising incidence of cigarette-related disease.

Thus, the suspicions about cigarettes and ill health, which began to emerge from the work of Raymond Pearl and Hammond and Horn, have been increasingly confirmed by a huge body of medical and scientific evidence, accepted by medical authorities in every developed country and acted on by many governments. Many countries have national laws regulating smoking and the promotion of smoking, and making smoking education part of the required curriculum in schools. Whole areas of these societies are now closed to smokers.

Smokers have become a shriveling and defensive minority, huddled into smoke-filled ghettos on airplanes and trains, barred from many public areas. Smoking has been identified

U.S. CIGARETTE CONSUMPTION DOWN

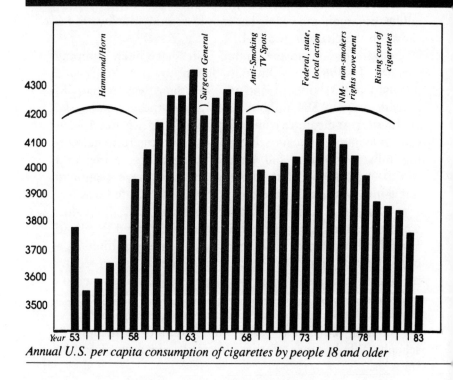

Annual U.S. per capita consumption of cigarettes by people 18 and older

Source: U.S. Department of Agriculture, 1983 estimate by OSH, DHHS

as a drug addiction by the American Psychiatric Association and by the National Institute for Drug Abuse.

All in all, in many developed countries, cigarette smoking is perceptibly on the way to becoming an activity restricted to consenting adults in private, and there is talk of a nonsmoking younger generation by the year 2000.

The effects of changed smoking behavior are becoming visible. For example, during the past thirty years, the tar and nicotine weighted sales average of all U.S. cigarettes has been dropping, and there have been corresponding improvements in health. Autopsy studies comparing smokers (who smoked the older high-tar/nicotine cigarettes) who died of causes other than lung cancer during 1955–1960 and smokers who died during 1970–1977 (who had to have smoked lower-tar/nicotine brands), showed far fewer damaging lung changes in the latter group. This has led to a prediction of lower lung-cancer death rates among cigarette smokers in the future.

A number of studies have also shown that long-term (ten years or more) use of filter-tipped cigarettes carries a lower risk of human lung cancer than does the continued smoking of nonfiltered cigarettes.

Long before the effects of ACS policies and actions in the smoking field began to become apparent, Richard Carter wrote:

> The society [ACS] must be credited with placing the conquest of cancer ahead of all other considerations in deciding to set its tobacco findings before the American public. Perhaps one should not applaud a voluntary health association for being devoted to health and being principled in that devotion; nobody hails a parent-teacher group for being interested in education. Yet, in the curiously cynical atmosphere of the contemporary United States, when voluntary health associations are discussed more for their fund-raising activities than their health contributions, rationality may be served by pointing out that the society decision to expose the hazards of smoking was courageous.

XI

The Cell Yields a Secret

Twelve sites of cancer account for about two-thirds of all cases of the disease in the United States, and 85 percent of deaths. But there have been significant changes in the death rates from several of these tumors during the past fifty years. In the 1930s, 1940s, and 1950s, the number one cancer killer of American women was cancer of the uterus, which included both the endometrium—the lining of the body of the womb—and the cervix or neck of the womb. In September 1926 Dr. James Ewing, a leading pathologist and one of the founders of the American Society for the Control of Cancer, spoke about the frustrations in treating cervical cancer: "[There are] no specific symptoms [to rely upon] for early diagnosis . . . [it] developes abruptly and advances to a serious condition in many cases in a few weeks or months." Dr. Ewing advocated "insistent" repair of all childbirth lesions, and repeated examinations—at least every six months.

The death rate for uterine cancer in America was above 30 per 100,000 women in 1930; today, it is about 8 per 100,000. A good part of this dramatic decline is due to the discovery in 1928, by research physician/scientist Dr. George N. Papanicolaou, that the uterus and the cervix shed cells in vaginal fluid, and that it was possible to diagnose cancer *in situ* from these cells. That is, cancer could be found more readily in the cervix than in the uterus itself—before it became a tumor. At this previsible stage, it is virtually 100 percent curable via a simple surgical technique.

76

That a cancer could be found this early, through the examination of cells (cytology), was a totally new idea. But like many original medical discoveries, Dr. Papanicolaou's astonishing finding was at first ignored and permitted to languish. It required the insight and courage of the American Cancer Society's director of medical and scientific research, Dr. Charles S. Cameron, to recognize and propagate it. He had valuable help from a young surgeon, Dr. Arthur I. Holleb, who many years later became the Society's senior vice-president for medical affairs.

The "Pap test," as it has come to be called, is now an integral part of medical practice, used worldwide for routine screening for cervical cancer. Its early history is largely unknown to today's practitioners and patients, but is worth exploring because it illustrates how important discoveries about cancer may come from research in unrelated areas—one of the justifications for much basic, seemingly impractical research. It also shows how a vital, potentially lifesaving discovery may remain unrecognized and undeveloped even by its discoverer; and how long it takes to create the technical support for a new test and to persuade the medical profession that the discovery is indeed useful.

George Papanicolaou was born in May 1883 in Kyme on the island of Euboea, Greece. His father, a physician, wanted his son George to become a doctor and practice with him. But after graduating from the University of Athens Medical School in 1904 and practicing with his father for a short time, the young Dr. Papanicolaou left to study biology with Dr. Ernst Haeckel in Munich, Germany. He also took a course in marine biology in Trieste during his Easter vacation.

After earning his Ph.D. in biology, he found no place to continue research in Greece, so he went to France and took a position at the newly established Marine Laboratories in Monaco. He had meanwhile met and married Mary Mavroyeni, the daughter of a colonel in the Greek Army.

Returning to serve in that in army during the Balkan War

of 1912–13, he heard from several soldiers of the opportunities in the United States and decided to emigrate. When George Papanicolaou and his wife sailed on the *Athenai* in 1913, they had little more than their tickets and the $250 in cash required for entrance by U.S. Immigration.

Papanicolaou was taken on as an assistant in anatomy at Cornell University, and his wife was hired as his laboratory aide. They began working on a problem that had interested him in Munich: sex determination. The subjects were guinea pigs. Dr. Papanicolaou published his first U.S. paper in *Science* in March 1915: "Sex Determination and Sex Control in Guinea Pigs." According to his biographer, Dr. E. Carmichael:

> Interested in continuing his work on sex determination, Dr. Papanicolaou stated, "I asked for the privilege of using some animals in order to test the theory of sex determination by x and y chromosomes in spermatozoa and ova." The experiments required obtaining the ova of the female guinea pigs at a precise state of development . . . while they were undergoing mitotic division with the formation of polar bodies, approximately at maturity but before the extrusion of the ova from the follicles. He knew that this stage of development occurred at about the time of ovulation. As their work proceeded, it became more and more evident that the existing notions of the period of ovulation in the guinea pig were of no practical value, or were actually incorrect. Apparent solutions to this problem were most unsatisfactory as they involved either the removal of the ovary by operation or sacrificing the animal [in effect ending the experiment].

The possible answer came to him one morning: "The females of all higher animals have a periodical vaginal menstrual discharge; so lower animals, such as the rodent, should also have one, but one probably too scanty to be evident externally." No thorough investigation of the estrus cycle of the guinea pig had been made, so Dr. Papanicolaou determined to do this. He bought a small nasal speculum (an instrument for enlarging the opening of a tube or canal) and began taking samples of guinea-pig vaginal discharge daily. These revealed that the animals did have a regular menstrual cycle, lasting twenty-four hours and recurring every fifteen to sixteen days. His vaginal smears revealed "an impressive wealth of diverse cell forms and a sequence of distinctive cytologic [cellular] patterns."

This knowledge enabled Papanicolaou to correlate the cellular changes with changes occurring in the ovary and uterus. His observations were reported in *Science* and in the *American Journal of Anatomy* in July and September 1917, the latter article coauthored by Papanicolaou's chairman, Dr. Charles Stockard. This fact led to Stockard's receiving credit for Papanicolaou's discovery. The latter was understandably chagrined. He spoke to Stockard, who assured him that never again would his name be attached to Papanicolaou's work. (Other researchers applied Papanicolaou's findings to the study of the rat, and this led to finding estrogenic hormones in the ovary, and eventually to Dr. George W. Comer's discovery of the luteal hormone, which plays an essential role in human fertility.)

In 1920 Dr. Papanicolaou began using his vaginal-smear technique to study human cells. At first he had only a single subject, whom he followed for twenty-one years because of the perfect regularity of her menstrual cycle; his wife, Mary.

Vaginal cytology in women was difficult; other investigators had tried it and had not found the changes seen in animals. In any case, not being a clinician, Dr. Papanicolaou had not been able to study cytology in groups of women. In 1925, however, the anatomy department of Cornell University established a working relationship with Women's Hospital of the City of New York. Through Dr. George Ward, director of Woman's Hospital, who was also a professor of gynecology at Cornell, Papanicolaou would have the opportunity to begin trying to delineate cyclic cytological changes in women as he had done in the guinea pig.

His twelve subjects were mainly hospital personnel, from whom he obtained daily vaginal smears for two to three months. He also studied several pregnant women. Based on these cases, he wrote a paper, "The Diagnosis of Early Human Pregnancy by the Vaginal Smear Method," published in 1925.

When he had established normal cytological changes, Dr. Papanicolaou began studying the cells of women with various pathologies. This led to the breakthrough. Says Carmichael, "It was inevitable that among these, some would have a genital malignancy." He quotes Papanicolaou: "The first observation of cancer cells in a smear of the uterine cervix was one of the most thrilling experiences of my scientific career."

Papanicolaou continued to study women who had genital cancer, and presented his findings in a paper titled "New Cancer Diagnosis" on January 4, 1928, at the Third Race Betterment Conference, in Battle Creek, Michigan. This was perhaps not the best forum he could have chosen—it was not a medical meeting—but the paper was perceived as news and received a headline; FINDS NEW CANCER DETECTION METHOD, in the *New York World* the next day.

Nonetheless, Dr. Papanicolaou said, it "failed to convince my colleagues of the practicability of this procedure." Leading pathologists believed that since the cervix was easily explored by biopsy, a relatively simple procedure, the cytological examination "appeared to be superfluous."

Gynecologists, Papanicolaou noted, were interested in structural (morphological) rather than cellular changes in the lining of the vagina and cervix in relation to menstrual cycles.

Since his own colleagues were not encouraging, he did not pursue his work in cancer diagnosis but directed his cytology studies toward endocrine changes. His next important paper, in 1933, was "The Sexual Cycle in the Human Female," detailing cellular changes during the reproductive cycle. His findings were valuable but not applicable to cancer diagnosis. Papanicolaou did not return to that field for ten years.

Dr. Stockard died and was replaced in 1939 as chairman of the anatomy department by Dr. Joseph Hinsey (who was also chairman of the Department of Physiology). Hinsey had been intrigued by Papanicolaou's 1928 report on cancer diagnosis, and thought that the work ought to be pursued. He urged Papanicolaou not to take a pharmaceutical company's grant of $4,000 to investigate the effects of androgen—a male hormone—on muscle tissue, but to get back to cellular diagnosis of uterine cancer.

Says Carmichael: "Dr. Papanicolaou expressed his previous discouragement and anxiety concerning the availability of sufficient funds and clinical material for the task. Dr. Hinsey promised his wholehearted support and together they outlined a program whereby 'the first step would be the development and establishment of its validity; the second would be to train others to use it: and finally, an effort would be made to educate the medical profession and the public [about the usefulness of the method].' "

Phase one was put into operation at New York Hospital: Every woman admitted to the gynecological service was required to have a routine vaginal smear taken. Slides were made using a fixative developed by Papanicolaou, and then stained and examined by him. Now came the second breakthrough: It soon became evident that "by use of the vaginal smear, a considerable number of asymptomatic and therefore unsuspected cases of uterine malignancy have been discovered, some of them in such an early stage of development that they were invisible to the unaided eye, or undemonstrable by the biopsy method," said Dr. Papanicolaou.

He and a gynecological pathologist, Dr. H. F. Traut, presented the findings in March 1941 to the New York Obstetrical Society in a report entitled "The Diagnostic Value of Vaginal Smears in Carcinoma of the Uterus." The physician who commented on the paper, Dr. I. C. Rubin, said, "If this proves diagnostic in a large number of cases of hidden type of carcinoma and of the early hitherto unrecognizable carcinoma of the cervix . . . then we have made a great advance in the armamentarium in this field." Dr. Hinsey noted that "the problem is different from tissue pathology [where] we have not only the cytology of the cells, but also the orientation of those cells in tissue." He likened the technique to that of diagnosing blood diseases from a blood smear. Dr. Papanicolaou was fifty-eight years old when the paper was published in the *American Journal of Obstetrics and Gynecology* later that year.

The Cornell group wanted to do more checking before certifying that the new method was ready for general use. Since this was a new technique and the cell changes indicating cancer were often subtle—not immediately apparent to those untrained in the technique—practitioners would need to know what to look for if cytological diagnosis was to become universally applicable. A skilled Japanese illustrator, H. Murayama, was added to the team to create a pictorial guide to cell changes. Because the United States was at war with Japan, the U.S. government required that two American doctors on the team be responsible for Mr. Muryama.

Two interesting cases of cancer diagnosed with the cellular technique were presented to the New York Medical Society in 1942. One was a sixty-one-year-old woman with chronic bladder problems. A vaginal smear suggested malignancy, but standard techniques (curettage and biopsies) did not confirm it. The woman continued to have positive smears for four months, but still only benign tissue was found. A later curettage did yield equivocal tissue that some pathologists read as benign, others as probably malignant. After a hysterectomy, a small cancer was detected behind a benign lesion (leiomyoma) in a corner of the uterus.

In another woman, the smear revealed cells thought to be squamous-cell carcinoma of the cervix, but careful examination revealed no visible changes, nor did repeated biopsies show any cancer. The woman was carefully watched for four months. Then a white spot in the epithelium turned out to be an early squamous cell cancer of the cervix.

As Dr. Carmichael observes, "Two important points were made: the vaginal smear permitted a diagnosis much earlier than would have been possible by biopsy, and the diagnosis would not have been made had routine vaginal smears of all patients not been taken."

By 1943 Dr. Papanicolaou and his team were ready to publish a monograph, "Diagnosis of Uterine Cancer by the Vaginal Smear," which had twenty-two pages of colored plates drawn by Mr. Murayama. So meticulous were these drawings that the size, shape, and staining reactions of abnormal cells were clearly visible. To achieve certain effects, the artist used brushes from which he had pulled all but a single hair.

The Cornell group's observations were confirmed by other investigators in New York and Boston. Nevertheless, most pathologists refused to accept cytological detection; they said it would not be possible to review the thousands of slides needed to screen a great many women for cancer.

XII

The Selling of the Cell

Like many novel ideas and techniques in medicine, cytology would have to be sold to doctors. It seemed to have importance in cancer, and the American Cancer Society was in a position to do something about it. The Society had begun its research program in 1945, and Dr. Charles S. Cameron, who became its director in 1946, was one of the first to see the possibilities of Papanicolaou's discovery.

"I was on the [surgical] staff of Memorial, and we were across the street from Cornell. The students would tell me about this guy who had discovered a test for early cancer of the uterus. And I got interested enough to go over and talk to him," Cameron said many years later.

He became a friend to the Greek researcher, who was somewhat isolated from the New York Hospital establishment.

He continued: "[As] a result of my conversations with Dr. Papanicolaou and discussion with people I regarded highly, like Howard Taylor [at Memorial] and Joe Meigs, who was doing superb work with Ruth Graham in Boston [Dr. Graham proved to Meigs, a surgeon, that cytology could find cancers even where the surgeon couldn't see them]. I got the idea that this was a great opportunity to save lives. So I pushed the Cancer Society for backing this full tilt. We put it in our publications for doctors and made much of it for the laymen in films and pamphlets. The cumulative effect was that it got under way faster than I think it otherwise would have."

Dr. Cameron persuaded the ACS to sponsor the First National Cytology Conference, at the Somerset Hotel in Boston in 1948. One hundred experts—half in favor of cytology, the rest doubters or opponents—were invited as guests by the Society. There was a lively debate for two days. "I think that perhaps did something to persuade people that it was here to stay," Dr. Cameron recalled in 1976.

A number of resolutions were adopted by the Cytology Conference. Perhaps the most important dealt with the need for criteria to determine whether cells were malignant and the need to train cytologists or cytopathologists to read and interpret cellular smears.

Now Papanicolaou's discovery had reached the critical point: It would require skillful timing and coordination to begin moving the test from the research laboratory to the clinic without alienating gynecologists and pathologists and without stimulating the public to demand tests that were not yet available.

Thus, the Cytology Conference agreed to avoid premature publicity about the test. Dr. Papanicolaou himself opposed an intensive campaign to encourage women to ask their doctors for smear examinations until a sufficient number of technicians and pathologists had been trained to interpret the slides correctly.

The experts decided that the new diagnostic method would be most effective if shared among clinicians who would take smears, cytologists and cytopathologists who would prepare and read slides, and tissue pathologists who would confirm the diagnosis with a biopsy examination. An Inter-Society Cytology Council was set up to assure that the three disciplines would cooperate. A secondary purpose was to keep cytology out of the hands of quacks, or untrained medical personnel.

There was a serious argument among pathologists over *in situ* cancer. Was it really cancer? This debate, which persists to this day, was recollected by Dr. Lewis Robbins, a well-known pathologist:

> The Pap smear isn't diagnosing cancer, it's diagnosing a precursor. Why do they call it cancer then? Because nobody would pay any attention if they called it dysplasia [abnormal tissue]. If you call it *carcinoma in situ*, then they will examine it, do something with it.
>
> I remember a battle royal at Roswell Park [Memorial Institute] in 1946. The pathologist was saying that the Pap smear is no good. One physician said *carcinoma in situ* is not cancer, but we have to call it cancer. The pathologist said we can't call it cancer if it doesn't metastasize or if it hasn't already metastasized. But we did.

In 1947 Dr. Arthur I. Holleb was honorably discharged with the grade of lieutenant from the navy, where he had been treating cancer patients in the Brooklyn Navy Hospital. He went to see Dr. Cameron, who had been his chief at that hospital and was now with the American Cancer Society. Holleb recalls:

> I was young and single, and I wanted to go back into surgical practice. Charlie Cameron said, "I want you to do something for the American Cancer Society." I said, "What's that?" And he said "There's this new thing called a Papanicolaou smear. I want you to travel round the country and sell this to pathologists and gynecologists. It could be useful in the early diagnosis of cancer of the cervix."
>
> It would be for nine months or a year. I said okay. First I got to know Dr. Papanicolaou, and learned about his work. Then I began making appointments to go to medical schools and clinics around the country to talk about the test. And I would visit divisions and units of the ACS, and tell them about it. I traveled on overnight trains, and on DC-3s; I'd make appointments with leading gynecologists and pathologists at medical centers. I got thrown out of more offices. . . .
>
> Gynecologists would say, "Don't bother me; if there is a

lesion, I can see it." And pathologists in those days, they wanted a formal biopsy. "Me look at cancer cells on a slide?" That was in the realm of exfoliative cytology, a science that was just barely beginning.

I guess the pathologists didn't want to be looking at a thousand or ten thousand slides to find one positive and all the rest negative. The suggestion was made that we would train technicians to read slides, that the pathologist would look only at questionable cells. This was a disturbing concept: technicians can't know pathology, only pathologists know pathology.

There were a few progressive-minded pathologists and gynecologists who saw the value of the Pap smear, but not too many. I don't think that I convinced anyone during my nine months. It was very frustrating back then. I think that Charlie Cameron deserves a great deal of credit, staying with cytology and putting it over.

There were many people in the Cancer Society medical group who were very skeptical of this. They said, "Even if it does diagnose early cancer, or cancer earlier than we can detect it at the present time it will also result in a lot of false positives [that is, finding abnormal cells where there is no disease], leading to unnecessary surgery. And since it will be radical surgery, there will be a sizable mortality, and we will kill more people than we will save." They could have been right, but the early experience indicated that that was not going to happen. Properly interpreted, the smear was quite accurate, in fact, it was finding cancers, very early tumors, that no other method could locate at the time.

Mainly the doctors were skeptical: The test was not going to work. It was entirely too simple. After all, those cells had been lying around for years. Why hadn't somebody found this before? The physicians thought this way, and they were fearful that we would educate the public to create a demand for which we could not supply the professional competence. But the laymen on the ACS board were all for it.

The medical people pointed out that there were not enough people who could interpret the smears correctly. So the ACS provided money for technicians to be trained by competent cytopathologists, of whom there were very few. And we made films for both lay people and physicians, to explain it. And we provided funds to Papanicolaou to continue his work.

Then we arranged that meeting in Boston in 1948, the first conference on cytology that had national importance, I believe.

And about a year later the Pap test began to take off. It was not just the meeting that did it, it was the fact that the Cancer Society got terribly interested in the Pap smear at that time. The money was rolling in, and we had the research commitment to spend at least twenty-five percent, and we had all those smart people who knew how to use modern communications techniques to back the program.

The Society's Medical and Scientific Committee said in 1951 that "in view of the poorly understood changes occurring in the uterine cervix, the Society will use its influence to procure a better understanding of the fundamental facts concerning carcinoma-in-situ, differential diagnosis of lesions simulating carcinoma-in-situ, and the clinical significance of the vaginal smear."

The Society's 1951 scientific meeting focused on exfoliative cytology, and Dr. Papanicolaou was given an ACS grant to investigate cytology in breast cancer. Dr. Cameron told the annual meeting of the Society, "We need not wait for more evidence; there is enough evidence on hand to justify taking the position—for women over forty, vaginal smear twice a year. Can we justify delaying any longer a vigorous campaign to press the use of the smear? My conscience and the opinion of those with the widest experience in its use say no."

By 1952 the Society had approved fifteen laboratories to train pathologists in exfoliative cytology. And the medical and scientific committee gave ACS divisions the authority to support the training of cytotechnicians locally in approved facilities.

Meanwhile, Dr. Papanicolaou and his associates had broadened the use of exfoliative cytology in diagnosing cancer not only of the cervix and endometrium but in the vagina and fallopian tubes. The technique had also been extended to examinations of urine, sputum, gastric washings, ascites (fluid from the peritoneal cavity), prostate secretions, spinal fluid, and breast secretions. A kidney cancer was found in one patient who had a consistent output of cancer cells in the urine but no lesion visible by X-ray. A fifty-year-old man with chronic bronchitis had abnormal cells in his sputum. X-rays and bronchoscopy revealed no tumor, but after the patient died, autopsy examination did find an *in situ* cancer in his lung.

Originally, Dr. Papanicolaou thought it might take three to six months to train a cytologist to read smears. But there were more nuances in cell changes than originally noticed: Papanicolaou classified them into five categories. Training in the technique of distinguishing the five subtle phases in cellular change would require a year. As a guide to cytologists, in 1948, Papanicolaou began work on a comprehensive *Atlas of Exfoliative Cytology*, with new drawings by Mr. Murayama. The book was produced in 1956 in loose-leaf format to permit adding new material.

The Pap test was accepted in a remarkably short time, and with a remarkable absence of feuding over turf. Carmichael states that "Dr. Papanicolaou credited Dr. Cameron with the foresight and careful planning which popularized the vaginal smear method in cancer diagnosis."

"The thing was timed pretty well," Dr. Cameron recalls. "It really dramatized the importance of early diagnosis in the treatment of cancer of the uterus. These women had been bleeding for years, the doctors were seeing all these advanced tumors, because there was no way to know what was going on until dysplasia or a tumor appeared. Now they could pick up cancer inside, not visible to the naked eye—they would not have known where to biopsy. So that was a tremendous advance. It certainly played a role in the reduction of deaths from cancer of the uterus."

Dr. Holleb credits the women of America with understanding the importance of early diagnosis, and demanding it. "You were supposed to tell your doctor you hadn't had a complete physical exam—underlining *complete*—if you hadn't had a Pap smear. Women did this. It was the power of American womanhood that ultimately sold the Papanicolaou smear, and helped to produce a seventy-percent reduction in deaths from cervical cancer in this country."

"Cytology was not the only factor in reducing the uterine-cancer death rate, of course," says Dr. Cameron. "Cuyler Hammond pointed out that the trend had started downward even before we had the Pap test. This resulted from a number of factors: We began to have more and better trained gynecologists. And you had a public that had been informed of the importance of abnormal bleeding. So you were seeing patients earlier, even without the smear. And there has been a great increase in the number of hysterectomies—obviously you are going to prevent cancers of the uterus if that organ has been removed before cancer has started, or avoid death from the disease if it's been taken out before invasion or metastasis."

By 1961, 30 percent of U.S. women had had at least one Pap test, according to a Gallup survey. In 1970 the number had risen to 53 percent, and in a 1973 survey by the National Center for Health Statistics, 75 percent of American females reported having had one or more Pap tests; 46 percent had had the examination within the past year.

Successful attempts have been made to persuade women to take their own smears. The main argument against it is that it may keep these women from getting complete pelvic examinations, but gynecologists have generally supported the idea. There has also been an effort to create automatic equipment to read slides. This has not as yet been successful.

According to Dr. Leopold Koss, chairman of the Department of Pathololology at Albert Einstein College of Medicine in New York City, widespread application of the Pap test was done "faster and probably better than the mass application of any new discovery. Don't forget that this was the first mass cancer-prevention program in the history of mankind. Regardless of how imperfect it might be, this is the first successful cancer-prevention program ever."

PAP TEST PREVENTS CANCER

When Dr. Koss made that statement, many experts were convinced that the Pap test had reduced deaths from cervical cancer. But there was no proof—mainly because this form of cancer has an average course of twenty years from the first *in situ* cells to death (in those comparatively few patients who die of the disease), and it is almost impossible to follow a large number of patients medically in the United States for that length of time.

Now, however, there is proof in a recent Swedish study that the Pap test not only saves lives but actually prevents cervical cancer. Sweden has population registries for every inhabitant. One action of the country has had a computerized registry of cervical-cancer screening for more than fifteen years that permitted researchers to follow a large population of women from all strata of society.

More than 90 percent of the women between ages thirty and fifty-nine in three Swedish counties, as well as 53 percent of those between sixty and sixty-nine and 25 percent of those above age seventy, were screened for cervical cancer by the Pap test during the ten years from 1971 to 1981. The group numbered 207,455 women, and their computerized Pap test and health records were the basis of the study. None of the women was lost to follow-up.

The results answer the question "whether Papanicolaou smears are effective in reducing the morbidity from cervical cancer in the population." The investigators state:

> The answer is clearly in the affirmative. When women are screened at least once, the incidence of cervical cancer drops from thirty-two in one hundred thousand to ten. . . . Among women with at least one normal smear, the incidence drops still lower to seven. There was a seventy-five-percent decrease in invasive cervical cancer incidence among women who had smears taken at least once during the ten-year period. Among

women who had never had smears taken, the incidence of invasive cervical cancer was four times as great as among those women who had been examined at least once.

If the entire population were completely screened, invasive cervical cancer cases would drop to between 1 and 5 per 100,000 women, the authors estimate. "The effectiveness of cervical cancer screening in reducing the morbidity or invasive cervical cancer is unequivocal."

In the United States, far fewer patients are dying of uterine cancer than before the Pap test. Currently, the overall five-year survival rate for cancer of the cervix is 65 percent. Cancer *in situ* detectable by the Pap test is virtually 100 percent curable: The cure rate for U.S. patients diagnosed with early cervical cancer is 80–90 percent. In endometrial (womb) cancer, survival averages 84 percent at all stages, 91 percent in early cancer, and virtually 100 percent for precancerous endometrial lesions.

Even those most skeptical of the value of early diagnosis credit part of this great increase in survival of patients with uterine cancer to the Pap test.

Exfoliative cytology has now been proved useful in screening high-risk groups for evidence of certain other cancers at an early stage:

Lung cancer: Sputum screening of uranium miners showed evidence of changes in epithelium (surface cells) inside lungs. When exposure to uranium continued, this developed into lung cancer. Hence, cytology is considered worthwhile in screening heavy smokers, asbestos workers, and others at high risk of lung cancer.

Bladder cancer: Examining urine can find asymptomatic cancer of the urinary bladder. It has proved practical to screen dye workers and others exposed to bladder carcinogens, and to follow patients treated for bladder cancer to seek early evidence of recurrence.

Gastric cancer: The incidence of this disease is so low in the United States that it is not considered cost-effective to do mass screening of gastric juices. However, in Japan, where the incidence of stomach cancer is high, mass screening by cytology has been effective in finding early, more curable cases.

Other sites: Cytology has been useful in finding cancers of the mouth, colon, and kidney, but not in detecting disease in asymptomatic cases.

XIII

Breast Cancer: Can Women Be Protected?

Among U.S. women, the cancer most feared is that of the breast. It presents the greatest threat—the disease attacks the breast more often than it does any other organ—and has offered until recently two main alternatives, both of them almost equally frightful to nearly all patients: a form of surgery that amounts to mutilation; or death. Until a year or two ago, the treatment generally considered most likely to cure breast cancer was some form of mastectomy, an operation that severs one or both breasts and very often includes removal of the surrounding lymph nodes and some muscles. For the great majority of women in our society, mastectomy means the destruction of their self-image, the loss of femininity.

For the past forty years, breast cancer has also been the leading cause of female cancer deaths in this country. It is now estimated that the number of American women dying of lung cancer has overtaken the number who die of breast cancer. However, breast cancer still leads other sites in incidence; there will be about 125,000 cases of the disease this year in American women as against about 50,000 cases of lung cancer.

One of eleven American women—about 9 percent—will develop breast cancer at some time in her life. The percentage has been mounting, since breast cancer is found increasingly often in women over age fifty, and the U.S. population

94

above that age has been growing. (The risk of breast cancer among American men is only about 1 percent that of women.) Currently, three women will be diagnosed for the disease every fifteen minutes; and in that same space of time, one will die of it. However, the death rate from this tumor has held steady despite the increased number of cases—probably because more and more cases are being diagnosed in the early, most curable stages.

The cause of breast cancer is not known, but certain risks have been identified. Women who have their first child after age thirty-five have three times the risk of breast cancer as those who have their first child by age eighteen. Early menarche (menstruation) or late menopause bear higher risks; women whose menopause starts at age fifty-five have twice the risk of those in whom menopause begins at age forty-five. Women whose mothers, sisters, or daughters developed breast cancer have three times the risk of the general population. In a recent study, women whose mothers and sisters both had breast cancer had fourteen times the risk of women in whose near relatives the disease has not appeared. Risk is also higher among women with certain other cancers (leukemia, uterine, colon, ovarian) or a preceding breast cancer. There is some reason to believe that a diet high in fat and protein may increase the risk of breast cancer, but this has not been proved. In sum, according to one cancer handbook, "there is increasing clinical, pathologic, and epidemiologic evidence that breast cancer is not a simple disease but an amalgam of adverse conditions."

How to reduce the toll of breast cancer? Wrote Dr. Arthur Holleb, senior vice-president for medical affairs at the American Cancer Society,

> Physicians engaged in the practice of oncology [cancer specialists] become more and more convinced that early detection and prompt treatment are directly responsible for cure or longer survival in many types of cancer.
> It is necessary to alert the public to the need for their

participation in finding more highly curable cancer, and breast
cancer is one of the more accessible sites.

Most specialists believe that finding and removing precancerous lesions in the breasts, or finding and treating breast
cancer at the earliest possible stage, before it has spread to
lymph nodes, offer the best assurance of avoiding or curing
the disease.

More than 90 percent of breast cancers are discovered by
patients: They have felt a lump, or seen some unusual skin
condition or nipple discharge, and reported it to their doctors.
However, in such cases, or in cases detected by physicians
during annual physical examinations, about 50 percent will
already show metastatic spread of the disease to axillary
(armpit) lymph nodes.

To try to detect breast cancer earlier, U.S. doctors developed a technique of examining breasts visually for external
signs of pathology, and by palpation for suspicious lumps.
There is no literature on the subject before the 1940s, but it
seems likely that Dr. Alfred Popma, a radiologist of Boise,
Idaho, then chairman of the Executive Committee of the
Idaho Division of the ACS (later national president), was one
of the first to teach patients how to examine their own breasts,
starting in 1938. The idea was for women to do this monthly,
so that they might find any early changes in their breasts,
rather than wait for annual physician examinations.

"We were seeing altogether too many cases of advanced
breast cancer," Dr. Popma said recently. "Women were finding their tumors, but didn't know what they had discovered,
or waited too long to report the symptom to their doctors."

In 1946 Dr. Popma used ACS volunteers to demonstrate
breast self-examination (BSE) to about 400 Idaho women in
workshops. These women told others, who began trying to
learn BSE from those who'd seen it demonstrated. "This
presented a certain hazard," Dr. Popma wrote, "because of
the sometimes incorrect interpretation of the method."

To teach more women the technique, Dr. Popma developed a slide presentation. But this didn't work well, and in 1947 he decided to make a film. "Many people thought this would be immoral, photographing a woman's breasts," Dr. Popma recalled. "They didn't think we could show it without creating trouble." But taking that risk to try to save lives seemed worthwhile.

Supported by the Idaho Division, Popma trained a local volunteer (she volunteered because her mother had died of breast cancer) to perform breast self-examination in front of a camera. The movie was shot with the help of a nurse and other female volunteers in 16mm color film at Dr. Popma's house. Then it was shown to an audience of Idaho women volunteers to find out if it would be acceptable. The twenty-one-minute training film was an immediate success. Fifteen prints were ready by January 1948, and Popma loaned several to the Texas ACS division, as well as Missouri, California, and other divisions.

The film was screened for several committees of the ACS National Board of Directors and approved by the board at a meeting in Philadelphia in June 1949. An observer at the meeting, Dr. Austin Diebert of the National Institutes of Health, was impressed and offered to pay half the cost of making a professional 35mm film in color and with a sound track. The ACS took him up, and thus began the first organized national program to teach women to protect themselves from breast cancer via self-examination. The film, featuring the well-known breast surgeon C. D. Haagensen of Columbia-Presbyterian Medical Center, was reviewed in glowing terms by the American Medical Association's journal in 1950. By the end of the year, 647 prints had been sold; and by 1953 more than 3 million American women had attended ACS screenings, at which there was always a doctor or nurse to answer questions.

However, palpation of the breast, and observation of surface changes, are relatively crude devices. Even the most sensitive medical fingers cannot feel a breast tumor less than one centimeter in diameter (about three-fifths of an inch), at which time it will have been growing for an average of nine years and may have already sent cancer cells on their metastatic voyage. And finding a bleeding nipple, or skin changes known as *peau d' orange* (pitted or dimpled skin, indicating underlying pathology), are not signs of early-stage cancer. Yet these were the best means available for detecting breast cancer until recent years.

Fortunately, researchers were working on better techniques. Since the discovery of X rays by Roentgen in 1895, radiologists had been trying to get clear images of soft tissues, and particularly of the living female breast. Dr. Stafford L. Warren of Strong Memorial Hospital in Rochester, New York, was the first to succeed, in 1930. But even though he was able to diagnose breast cancers with X rays, his work was not immediately followed up, mainly because surgeons at that time thought that palpation was all they needed.

A Philadelphia radiologist, Dr. Jacob Gershon-Cohen, took up the challenge of X-raying the breast and greatly refined and advanced the technique. It is now known as mammography, and Dr. Gershon-Cohen is considered one of its main developers. As early as 1937 he had advocated mammography examinations to screen women who had no symptoms for early detection of breast cancer, but he was almost alone in his advocacy.

In 1956 Gershon-Cohen and associates began a five-year screening program at Albert Einstein Medical Center in Philadelphia. During this five-year period, 1,312 women with no breast symptoms were given physical examinations and their medical histories were recorded. Mammograms were taken every six months. Ninety-two benign lesions were found, all correctly diagnosed by the radiologist from the X rays. Twenty-three seemingly malignant lesions were detected. Thirteen of these were identified as definitely malignant by Gerhon-Cohen, nine as probably malignant. There was only one false positive diagnosis; all of the rest were confirmed by biopsy examinations.

This was a phenomenal demonstration, but again the method was generally ignored—probably because other radiologists couldn't duplicate Gershon-Cohen's technique. He was extremely skillful and had special equipment others couldn't afford (he was wealthy, with a lucrative private practice). Most radiologists were unable to get clear pictures of the breast.

Dr. Robert Egan of M. D. Anderson Hospital and Tumor Institute in Houston, Texas, tried to do mammography, using Gershon-Cohen's techniques, without success. So he built his own equipment and used industrial film to get breast pictures accurate enough to diagnose cancer before biopsy. Egan was ridiculed by colleagues who still believed that soft tissues could be not be X-rayed. However, encouraged by the chief of surgery as well as the head of radiology, he doggedly continued his work. When he had X-rayed 1,000 women, among whom he correctly diagnosed 238 out of 240 cancerous tumors, he published his results. From that point on, mammography began to be widely accepted. Egan's technique proved reproducible and accurate. Radiologists could be trained in five days to do mammograms by his method, and a national comparative study among different institutions showed that the results were uniform.

In 1964 at least five physicians who either had been or were to become American Cancer Society presidents were involved in proving the reliability of mammography: Thomas Carlile, Murray Copeland, Warren Cole, Wendell Scott, and David Wood. Later, when Carlile, a radiologist, became ACS president, he and Dr. Copeland, a surgeon, helped persuade the American College of Radiology (ACR) to appoint an ad hoc committee to evaluate mammography. The ACR chairman, Dr. Present, said, "There are no great disagreements about skin dosage or about techniques of mammography; mammography contributes to cancer control and has the potential of reducing the death rate of cancer of the breast."

In 1963 Dr. Philip Strax, head of the Guttman Institute in New York City, created a screening program to assess breast-cancer detection by mammography. Enrolled in this study, were 62,000 women between the ages of forty and sixty-four, who were members of the Health Insurance Plan (HIP) of Greater New York. Randomly selected to enter a control group, which was not screened, or the study group, which was given clinical examinations and mammography, the women were checked at intervals during the next five years. At the end of that time, the study directors—Dr. Strax and HIP statistician Sam Shapiro—discovered that women over age fifty in the study group had suffered one-third fewer breast-cancer deaths than those in the control group. There was no statistical difference between the two groups below age fifty. After the study had gone on for seven years, the total number of cancers was nearly the same in both groups, but there were 108 breast-cancer deaths in the control group as against only 70 in the study group. At fifteen years of follow-up, this difference in cancer mortality persisted for women over age fifty.

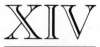

XIV

Breast X-Ray: Can It Save Lives?

In 1971 Dr. Strax suggested to Dr. Arthur Holleb, who had become the senior vice-president for medical affairs of the American Cancer Society, that the Society look at mammography as a screening device for breast cancer in women who had no symptoms. Dr. Holleb thought there might be some added benefit of earlier detection from the new technique.

The ACS appointed a breast-cancer task force made up of seventy of the leading experts in radiology, surgery, gynecology, and other pertinent specialties. They presented a program to the Society's board of directors to establish a dozen breast-cancer-detection demonstration projects (BCDDP) that would provide free clinics to take a medical history and give clinical, radiographic (mammographic), and thermographic (study of skin hot spots as possible clues to underlying pathology) examinations. According to Holleb, these four modalities were considered the "most effective program for earlier detection then available." Each clinic would screen 5,000 asymptomatic women annually for two years. In addition, existing breast-cancer clinics would be expanded. Dr. Holleb wrote later:

> The American Cancer Society deems it part of our stewardship
> to advance useful new diagnostic and detection techniques.
> The demonstration project was designed to find out if modern
> screening, including the teaching of breast self-examination, a

101

clinical breast examination, a mammogram and a thermogram, in a variety of community institutions—such as university centers, major hospitals, smaller community facilities, specialized institutions—could discover unsuspected early and readily curable breast cancer. Ancillary questions were whether qualified institutions, and highly specialized radiologists, would participate; and whether enough [asymptomatic] women would volunteer and faithfully return for annual follow-up examinations.

The original ACS plan for twelve two-year clinics was to cost about $1 million per year; the ACS Board of Directors was asked to vote the money.

It did so in 1972. Soon after that, the National Cancer Institute budget—greatly enlarged under the National Cancer Act of 1971—added funds for its cancer-control program. Holleb and Alan Davis, ACS vice-president, science editor, and Washington liaison, approached Dr. Frank J. Rauscher, director of NCI, with the proposal that the latter organization join in the project. Dr. John C. Bailar III, NCI's acting director of cancer control, was "totally disinterested and wanted no part of it, although no reason was given," according to Holleb. In view of Dr. Bailar's later statements, it is interesting that the record does not reveal any concern on his part in 1972 with putative risks of radiation.

His superior, Dr. Rauscher, seemed to want to cooperate in the demonstration projects. Yet after a series of meetings, he had not made up his mind. "It was exasperating," Holleb recalled later. "Finally I asked Dick [Rauscher] if he wanted to join us, or whether we should move ahead on our own. He wanted to know why we thought it was a good idea to expand the project, and we told him: the increasing risk of breast cancer in an aging population, the Strax study showing undeniable saving of lives, and hoped-for better results since mammography had been much improved since the HIP study. And he agreed."

The general policy worked out was that the NCI would put up 75–80 percent of the cost; the ACS would keep the cost low by supplying volunteer recruiters, secretaries, and other personnel, as well as expertise to the detection centers. With NCI help, the number of centers was tentatively enlarged to twenty; and the ACS began screening applications from institutions who wanted to set up breast-cancer-detection demonstration projects. They passed on recommendations to NCI for funding the BCDDP. The review officer at NCI, Dr. Nathaniel Berlin, was very supportive, according to Holleb, whereas Dr. Bailar—whose cancer-control branch would be ultimately responsible for NCI participation in the projects—continued to be uninterested.

The number of projects was expanded finally to twenty-nine at twenty-seven medical centers. Beginning in 1973, each would register, and examine by the four modalities, 10,000 asymptomatic women between the ages of thirty-five and seventy-four, and follow them for five years. Although Strax's study has shown no lifesaving benefit under age fifty, the radiological experts who set guidelines for the BCDDP thought that younger women should have the benefit of mammography screening. Their rationale: Breast cancer begins to be a significant threat to women at age thirty-five, and mammography had been considerably refined; it was able to produce much clearer images (more difficult in younger than older women) than those at the time of the Strax study, which had started some thirteen years earlier. Furthermore, the exposure to X rays in mammography had been sharply reduced, from an average of 6.4 rads in the Strax study to about one rad in the early 1970s. A new, alternative form of mammography was also to be tried—xeroradiography, which produces a positive image on paper, rather than the film negative created by standard X-ray equipment, and might pick up more or different suspicious lesions.

The ACS went all out to publicize the projects, and as a result tens of thousands of women registered. Then two very well-known women—Margaretta ("Happy") Rockefeller, wife of New York's Governor Nelson Rockefeller, and Betty

Ford, wife of President Gerald Ford—were operated on for breast cancer in 1975. Both women were open and candid about their experiences, and other women were suddenly made very aware of breast cancer. The BCDDP were immediately oversubscribed.

Although these were to be demonstration projects (with no control group; the Strax study, a clinical investigation, had had a control group), it was decided that much of clinical value might be learned from them. The NCI therefore funded a statistical center in Philadelphia to keep track of the registrants and findings. The BCDDP clinics began giving tens of thousands of breast examinations in 1973.

"Unexpectedly, the widespread use of mammography of asymptomatic American women in the BCDDP resulted in a controversy that polarized opinions to such an extent that the future of mammography was in jeopardy," wrote two professors of radiology at the University of California, Los Angeles, nearly a decade later.

The controversy started with a single individual. Dr. Bailar had been moved from his job as acting director of the cancer-control program at the NCI and appointed editor of the *Journal of the National Cancer Institute*. As a biostatistician, he became troubled about the possible risks of radiation used in mammography, and worried about its use to screen women under age fifty.

He asked for an interview with Dr. Rauscher to discuss these theoretical risks, and in October 1975 he met with Rauscher and other NCI officials, as well as ACS representatives. His analysis of the HIP study showed less benefit attributable to mammography than others had seen. And his study of radiation risks led him to believe that there were grave dangers in using mammography to screen younger asymptomatic women (as distinct from its use as a diagnostic tool in women of any age with symptoms). His assessment, published the following year in a medical journal, ended by saying, "I regretfully conclude that there seems to be a possibility that the routine use of mammography in screening asymptomatic women may eventually take as many lives as it saves. . . . Screening by medical history and physical examination alone will probably provide much or more of the same benefit without risk from irradiation, at least in women under some fairly high age limit."

Dr. Rauscher appointed three experts to estimate benefits of mammography in the HIP study, and to consider and estimate radiation risks and examine the pathology of the cancers found in the HIP study.

Meanwhile, Bailar began publicly protesting that radiation mammography was being unnecessarily used for screening in the BCDDP, which, he said (basing himself on a 1972 National Academy of Sciences report), might cause six cancers in every million women exposed to one rad each. He told journalists that "the [BCDDP] program contains seeds of a major disaster."

This coming from the editor of a prestigious cancer journal published by the NCI, was incendiary. Few if any reporters bothered to check, but accepted Bailar's warning as valid.

Actually, there were no studies showing hazard from radiation at anywhere near the low levels in BCDDP mammography. To achieve his estimate, Bailar had extrapolated from three studies of women—most of them under age twenty-five, when X-ray is most risky—who had been exposed to massive amounts of radiation: Japanese women who at age ten and above had survived huge doses of whole-body radiation from the atomic bombs at Hiroshima and Nagasaki; young Canadian and American women who had had multiple fluoroscopies of the chest during tuberculosis treatment; and young Canadian and American women treated with radiation for inflammation of the breast after giving birth. The NAS and Bailar had assumed a straightline risk—i.e., that the risk of all women exposed to any X-ray was proportional to the risks of those three young high-exposure groups. That, in other words, there was no level of radiation without risk.

Dr. Arthur Upton, one of the three experts appointed by

Rauscher, studied the same data for the NCI. He, too, supported the concept of a linear risk. Dr. Upton said that a single one-rad mammography examination would increase a thirty-five-year-old woman's risk of breast cancer by 1 percent per year. This sounded ominous, but what it meant was that since the normal risk of all women for breast cancer was then 7 percent, a mammogram might raise it to 7.01 percent, with decreasing risk for subsequent mammograms as time went by.

In an examination of the same data that Dr. Bailar, Dr. Upton, and the NAS had relied on, the National Cancer Institute pointed out:

> [While] recent epidemiologic studies suggest that X-ray doses generally greater than 100 rads may induce breast cancer in women after a 10–15 year latency period . . . there is no direct evidence that radiation levels utilized in mammography in the NCI-ACS detection program [one rad] can cause breast cancer in women. The levels of radiation in the detection program are 100- to 500-fold lower than those reported to have caused cancer in the studies cited above.

However, Bailar's ominous warnings had quickly become national TV and radio news, front-page stories and editorials. The effect on American women was immediate and devastating: The very basic distinction between mammography as a diagnostic tool for patients with breast symptoms and as a screening device for asymptomatic women was overlooked in popular discussions. Mammography, already established as a vital diagnostic tool, was being shunned by the public. Surgeons and radiologists from all over the country reported that women with symptoms were canceling appointments for mammography exams.

"These were women who needed mammograms, their surgeons needed the pictures because they were going to operate. Patients were staying away in droves," Dr. Holleb told a reporter on the CBS Television Network. "It's almost a panic kind of reaction, which is so terribly unfortunate."

Overlooked in most popular reports was the fact that in

the first year of the BCDDP, 262,276 women were screened, 5,000 biopsies were performed on the basis of clinic findings, and nearly 1,250 breast cancers (twice the expected number) were diagnosed and treated. Said leading breast-cancer surgeon Benjamin F. Byrd, Jr., clinical professor of surgery at Vanderbilt University and Meharry Medical College (and later president of the ACS): "To physicians, these figures meant that active screening was picking up hundreds of cancers that probably would not have been detected in the normal course of events for another year or two or three." Thus, it seemed that the BCDDP were showing that it would be possible to reduce the death rate from breast cancer.

In the CBS interview, Dr. Holleb said that even though the HIP study had found no reduced mortality from mammography screening in women between ages thirty-five and fifty, there were many below that age who might benefit: those at higher risk due to the various factors outlined in the previous chapter. "Between thirty-five and fifty," Dr. Holleb said, "the vast majority of women fall into this category that requires mammography examination in the hope of finding breast cancer early and reducing the unchanging mortality rate."

The media were unrelenting, however. Mammography became transformed almost overnight in the public's mind from a desirable examination into an unacceptable menace. In the BCDDP's the number of women examined monthly dropped from 24,000 before July 1976 to 17,000 afterward.

The National Cancer Institute and the ACS set up new guidelines for the demonstration projects in August 1976: Based on a study of the HIP project by Dr. Lester Breslow, mammography for routine screening of women under age fifty would be discontinued: radiation exposure of those fifty and older would be confined to less than one rad per examination; and informed-consent forms for women in the BCDDP would include more information on radiation risks. But these changes did not still criticism.

XV

"Purposeless Mutilations"?

The next round of troubles began when the NCI created a working group of "carefully chosen experts" under Dr. Oliver Beahrs of the Mayo Clinic to "ascertain what scientific information could be obtained from the BCDDP that could reflect possible gains achieved in the current use of mammography in screening for breast cancer."

Based on a preliminary report from the BCDDP management center, on May 3, 1977, the NCI changed the guidelines again, allowing certain exceptions in younger women:

> For all women 35 through 49 years of age (current age), routine annual screening by mammography will be discontinued except for the following situations:
> (a) A personal history of breast cancer.
> (b) A history of breast cancer in the screenee's immediate family (mother/sisters).

In an editorial entitled "Mammography Muddle," on May 12, the *New York Times* stated that "the Cancer Society is expected to acquiesce [to the new guidelines] but still contends that X-rays are beneficial for women over 35." The editorial referred to the BCDDP as a "dubious project" and said that "evidence is accumulating that the program may actually do more harm than good; the X-rays may conceivably cause cancer in a small number of otherwise healthy women." It accused the Cancer Society, "a politically powerful philanthopic organization," of letting "its zeal for combating cancer blind it to possible adverse consequences."

108

Dr. Holleb pointed out in a letter to the *Times* that the original BCDDP guidelines had been set by a committee of "nationally recognized physicians and scientists," and that experts in radiology, including those from the HIP study, had recommended "that women between thirty-five and seventy-four be included." Mammography had been much improved in clarity he said, and radiation had been reduced to about one-sixth or one-seventh of that used in the HIP study, making comparisons illogical as to both effectiveness and safety.

"More than 2,000 unsuspected breast cancers have been found among the 280,000 women in the projects to date [June 1977]," Dr. Holleb continued. "About 45 percent of those detected in screening have been found by *mammography alone*—i.e., physical examination showed nothing suspicious. About 30 percent of all breast cancers have been found in women under the age of 50, and in that group *mammography alone* led to 40 percent of the diagnoses."

What appeared as important clinical progress to breast-cancer physicians did not persuade critical biostatisticians—the latter reiterated that since there was no control group, the BCDDP were not a scientific experiment; therefore it could not be assumed that earlier detection would save lives.

The press took most of its cues from the critics. Irwin Bross, Ph.D., an epidemiologist at Roswell Park Memorial Institute, published an article with an associate in the *Journal of the American Medical Association* to the effect that diagnostic X-rays of any kind, even at very low levels of exposure, were causing leukemia and other diseases in the children of people who had been exposed.

Even before his article appeared, Bross had begun issuing statements attacking the ACS and BCDDP. Bross, whose accusations were widely disseminated by wire services, radio, and TV, said, "This exposure [in BCDDP] to diagnostic X-ray will probably result in the worst iatrogenic [caused by medical treatment] epidemic of breast cancer in history."

Bross continued to repeat his charge, and the ACS issued a statement some months later denouncing it as "false and unsubstantiated." It may have been the strongest rebuttal ever issued by the American Cancer Society. Its breast cancer demonstration project, carefully designed to search for a means of earlier diagnosis, and thereby to reduce the death rate from breast cancer, had become a threat to the society's integrity. More, the hopes that mammography might be useful in saving lives had somehow been transformed into an attack on the technique, not only in screening but in diagnosis of symptomatic patients, where it had been well established.

Even worse was to come. In September 1977 a preliminary report by a pathology subcommittee of the Beahrs working group, headed by Dr. Robert W. McDivitt of the University of Utah, stated that sixty-six women diagnosed for cancer in the BCDDP had been subjected to unnecessary mastectomies; their lesions were found by the subcommittee to be benign.

The *New York Times* commented editorially—under the headline MAMMOGRAPHY MISTAKE—that "women had their breasts wholly or partly removed because of erroneous diagnoses of cancer. . . . later determined to be benign. . . . Those who promoted the screening program were so certain of its value that they failed to design a research program to substantiate their theory."

This would seem to drive the final nail into the BCDDP. If women were being misdiagnosed and mutilated, something must be gravely wrong with the project. It did not help much that Dr. Holleb told the *Times* that "pathology is not part of the screening projects, nor of mammography." Indeed, pathology was used by the hospitals to ascertain whether a suspicious area picked up in the BCDDP was or was not cancer. Some critics were saying that finding such early tumors and *in situ* cancers only created problems that pathologists were not equipped to solve.

There was some good news, but it was intraprofessional,

not calculated to make headlines. *Medical World News* reported, "The mammography war isn't over. Radiologists are counterattacking with reports of stunning reductions in X-ray dosage to the surface of the breast. . . . New calculations suggest the amount of radiation reaching the center of the breast has been largely overestimated in the past." The report was based on information from Dr. Wende W. Logan, a consultant to Roswell Park Memorial Institute. Dr. Logan said that sharp pictures of the breast could be obtained with commercial equipment giving only about a third of a rad for each view, and that radiation at the midbreast was only about 5 percent of that to the skin, instead of the 25 percent previously calculated. Dr. Bailar was skeptical of Dr. Logan's claims, although they were verified by a Sloan-Kettering radiation physicist. Bailar did acknowledge that mammography radiation doses were "descending at a remarkably fast clip."

The following August (1978), the NCI's working group reported (but their report was not immediately released) that they had found diagnoses of the larger tumors in BCDDP so accurate that they had confined their pathological analysis to 506 that were less than one centimeter in diameter. These were the kinds of tumors the projects had hoped to find, the kind that offered the best chance of cure. Tumors of this size could be picked up only in mammograms. In that report, the sixty-six widely reported cases of incorrect tissue diagnosis had shrunk to forty-eight.

Even forty-eight unnecessary mastectomies—linked as they were to the BCDDP—were unacceptable, of course, if the subcommittee was correct. In the *Washington Post*, Daniel S. Greenberg assumed that it was. He reported that Dr. McDivitt's group "took the position that purposeless mutilation had been inflicted on many women."

Greenberg noted that a group of surgeons and other clinicians had disputed the McDivitt group and that this argument had held up the Beahrs committee's report for six months. He called it a "sorry business" and referred to the "cancer screening debacle," saying it "traces back to the American Cancer Society, which feasts on terrorizing the public about a dread disease." Greenberg charged that "many mastectomies were swiftly performed" on the basis of "minuscule lesions" with which "few of the pathologists in the screening program had any experience. . . . The mutilations were the outcome of medicine's gung-ho drive to deploy new diagnostic technologies long before any careful assessment has been made of their safety and reliability."

As it turned out, Greenberg's accusations were grounded in misinformation. About nine months earlier, *Medical World News* had reported that the McDivitt committee's analyses were largely based on the "wrong slides" of tissues taken from the patient's other (healthy) breast or from "representative" slides that did not include those with cancer cells. The magazine said that "the hospitals had preferred to keep their original slides" rather than turn them over to McDivitt's group.

As one example, said the magazine, at an Oakland, California, hospital, five cases had been reclassified by McDivitt's group as benign. All five were re-reviewed by the hospital's pathologists and outside pathologists, according to Dr. Robert Schweitzer, and "They all agreed, there's not one doubtful one among them. They're all cancer. So Dr. McDivitt didn't get the right slides? he was asked. 'Yes, that's right.' "

When the NCI's Beahrs working-group report came out in 1978, the original sixty-six cases questioned by McDivitt's subcommittee had become (by their count) sixty-four: Two had been incorrectly included because of computer error.

Of the sixty-four, eleven had been treated with only biopsies or segmental resections for diagnosis, not mastectomy, leaving fifty-three actual mastectomies.

Of the fifty-three, the pathology re-review confirmed eleven as cancer.

This left forty-two cases. Five were reclassified as "borderline," reflecting differences in interpretation among experts. This happens frequently in pathology, no matter how the cases are detected, since the change from normal to cancerous tissue is a continuum, and thus it is a matter of judgment at which point the change actually takes place.

Of the thirty-seven remaining cases, twenty-nine had had mastectomies in two-stage operations. That is, a biopsy was first obtained, and then, after consultations and consideration of options, surgery was performed from one to 113 days later. None was done "swiftly." Pathologists and surgeons had followed the same procedures most often used by responsible professionals in such cases.

In the eight cases that remained, surgery was performed in one stage: First a tissue biopsy was taken; it was confirmed as cancer in seven of the cases by the hospital pathologist; and mastectomy followed on the same day. In one instance the patient had had cancer treatment in one breast and had elected surgery for the other. Reviewing these cases, the project pathologist classified four as not being cancer.

The Beahrs working-group report concluded that rather than numerous mistakes in diagnosis and treatment, "great care was given to the diagnosis and management of the women who had possible breast cancer or significant pathologic changes . . . in almost all instances the treatment, based on information which the medical record indicates was available to the surgeon at the time of management, was consistent with accepted surgical practice."

None of this information, which almost entirely contradicted the original charges about sixty-six misdiagnoses and "mutilations," made front-page news or the evening telecasts.

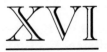

XVI

Developing a Clearer Picture

The Beahrs working group recommended that the BCDDP be continued through five annual screenings, and that

> reduced-dose film mammography (or xeroradiography) be continued as a routine screening modality for:
>
> (a) All women 50 years of age and older
>
> (b) Women at ages 40–49, only when they have a personal history of breast cancer or a history of breast cancer in first-degree relatives (mothers or sisters)
>
> (c) Women at ages 35–39, only when they have a personal history of breast cancer.

Although the original group of 275,000 BCDDP participants shrank during the five years of the project to 171,000, Dr. Larry H. Baker, chairman of the BCDDP Data Management Group, considered it "remarkable that, regardless of age, more than half the women who entered the program attended all five screenings."

The projects went forward to their scheduled completion.

In 1980, the ACS revised all of its suggested general cancer-checkup guidelines for physicians. At that time they recommended that "women over 50 should have a mammogram every year." A 1982 summary of the full five-year results by the BCDDP Management Group stated:

> "Of the 4,443 cancers recorded in the BCDDP population, more than 80 percent were detected by the 29 centers. Approxi-

mately one-third (32.4 percent) of the 1,557 cancers detected by the centers were smaller cancers, either noninfiltrating or infiltrating cancers (< 1 cm). More than 80 percent of all cancers detected showed no evidence of nodal involvement. Although there is no preselected comparison group, it is clear that a high proportion of cancers detected within the BCDDP are localized and according to tumor registry data, these patients should have an excellent prognosis.

Physical examination and mammography both contributed cases not detected by the other, but the contribution of mammography was substantially greater. The relative contribution of mammography alone (in the absence of positive physical findings) was 41.6 percent compared with 8.7 percent for physical examinations (in the absence of positive mammogram findings). This relative contribution of mammography was impressively high in the detection of smaller cancers—49 percent for noninfiltrating cancers and 52.6 percent for infiltrating cancers (< 1 cm).

The relative contribution of mammography was also impressively higher than had been shown in previous reports. . . ."

In 1983 the board of directors of the American Cancer Society concluded:

Recently reported results from the American Cancer Society–National Cancer Institute Breast Cancer Detection Demonstration Projects indicate that one-third of the breast cancers occurred in women between the ages of 35 and 49 years, and most of these lesions were either *in situ* or did not involve regional lymph nodes. Most of the cancers were detected by mammography and a much higher percentage were detected by mammography alone than by physical examination alone.

Because of the detection of some palpable and small breast cancers and because of the reduced radiation exposures now possible with optimum mammographic technique and carefully monitored equipment, a favorable benefit/risk ratio can be expected in women beginning at age 40 and older.

Perhaps partly as a result of the intense scrutiny of the BCDDP, and American women's concern about risks of radiation, mammography continued to be refined and improved during the 1970s. Radiation dosages were lowered, images sharpened. And the terror and confusion engendered by the "mammography war" began to recede. In 1983 Dr. Gerald D. Dodd, professor and chairman of radiology at the University of Texas Cancer Center, Houston, was able to report to the ACS National Conference on Breast Cancer:

> The criticism of mammography as a diagnostic and/or survey procedure has decreased, primarily due to the perception that there has been an increase in quality and a concomitant decrease in risk. . . . The results of the examination of 280,000 women in the Breast Cancer Detection Demonstration Project support this conclusion. . . . It is reasonable to conclude that the potential benefits of mammography far outweigh the minimal risk incurred by the examination.

At the same conference, Dr. Philip Strax, who had become clinical professor of oncology at the University of Miami (Florida) School of Medicine, said:

> The serious import of breast cancer lies in its potential for metastatic spread, which probably starts early in the course of the disease. Detection of the lesion when immunocompetence [the body's immune system] can control the metastases leads to long-term survival. . . .
>
> The threat posed by breast cancer to women is greater than ever. The increasing incidence plus the increasing tendency for it to become manifest in women younger than 35 years of age make methods for control urgent. The only proven means to do this is mass screening. However, a new risk has been introduced, i.e., the risk of not using our best and perhaps only means to detect the disease before it becomes palpable and when it is most curable. Concern over radiation risk in mammography by preventing its use can undo our efforts to reduce mortality. It has been widely demonstrated that the radiation risk of modern mammography is negligible, if there is any, particularly in women older than 30 years of age, for whom mass screening is indicated.

Also in 1983, the ACS recommended that the Cancer-Related Checkup Guidelines for mammography in breast-cancer detection be broadened: All women who have reached age thirty-five should have a baseline mammogram for later comparison. Asymptomatic women age forty to forty-nine ought to have a physical examination of the breasts annually, and mammography at intervals of one to two years.

In 1984 the American Medical Association's Council on Scientific Affairs suggested that women should have their first mammographic examination between the ages of thirty-five and forty. And during their forties, mammograms were recommended at one- to two-year intervals.

More recently, many newspapers and magazines have abandoned their criticisms of mammography and have begun to advocate it as a means of saving more lives from breast cancer.

PART THREE

Cancer Research

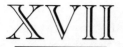

XVII

Cancer Research: The Black Hole

Organized cancer research did not really exist until the twentieth century. Before then, what had been learned about malignancies came largely from clinical observation and from scientific and clinical investigations into other diseases.

Starting around 1900, various committees and institutes were founded for research targeted at cancer: in England (Imperial Cancer Research Fund) and Germany (Institute for Cancer Research) and others in Denmark, Sweden, and Switzerland. In the United States the lead was taken in 1901 by New York State, whose legislature voted a cancer-research grant to Dr. Roswell Park of Buffalo. The seed grant to Dr. Park grew into the present Roswell Park Memorial Institute, one of the world's leading cancer centers. Other cancer research was started early in the century at the New York Skin and Cancer Hospital, Memorial Hospital, and Columbia University, all in New York City. The American Association for Cancer Research was founded in 1907. It urged the publication of demographic material relevant to cancer incidence and mortality.

When the American Society for the Control of Cancer (ASCC) was founded in 1913, cancer was not seen as an urgent health priority. The leading causes of death in the United States were heart disease, tuberculosis, and pneumonia/influenza; cancer was seventh on the list. Dr. Frederick L. Hoffman, a statistician at Prudential Life Insurance Company

121

of America, was the first to spot an ominous change: "I am absolutely convinced that the cancer death rate is increasing and the larger recorded mortality is not primarily due to unproved medical diagnosis and more accurate methods of death certification," he told the 1913 meeting of the American Gynecological Society.

The ASCC founders did not include cancer research in their agenda; Dr. Howard Taylor wrote thirty years later, "Our Society was founded for lay education . . . cancer research, in fact, was intentionally omitted." However, Dr. Taylor must have limited his definition of *research* to the basic sciences and clinical investigations. A year after the Society was founded, it had an active Statistical Advisory Committee chaired by Dr. Hoffman. Its purpose: to lay the foundations for epidemiological research. The committee suggested to the director of the United States census that cancer be included in the government's annual volume on mortality statistics; as a result, the director of the census authorized the first official U.S. monograph on cancer mortality in 1914. But that was all that the government provided in cancer-mortality information until 1925. Meanwhile, the ASCC was the only regular source of such data; then the Public Health Service took on the responsibility.

The National Cancer Act of 1937 had established the National Cancer Institute, the first of the National Institutes of Health, to "conduct researches, investigations, experiments and studies relating to the causes, diagnosis and treatment of cancer; assisting and fostering similar research activities by other agencies, public and private . . ." But the NCI cancer-research budget was tiny. Biomedical cancer research was widely scattered and only minimally funded when Mrs. Lasker insisted, in 1944, that the American Cancer Society devote 25 percent of its budget to research.

When the ACS began its biomedical research program in 1945, it encouraged what is known as investigator-initiated research. That is, medical and scientific investigators submit proposals to the Society for projects they wish to undertake, and the Society funds those it deems most worthy. To assure objectivity in judging the value of proposed projects, the abilities and training of applicants and the integrity of their institutions, for the first few years of its research program the ACS turned to the National Research Council (NRC) of the National Academy of Sciences, an independent organization.

The American Cancer Society began funding biomedical research at a time when cancer was generally considered to be an unsolvable enigma. Cancer research had been a black hole, avoided by most biomedical scientists. The NRC set up a Committee on Growth, a title deemed broad enough to cover all the disciplines which might bear on cancer. The committee was made up of recognized experts in the various sciences. It began its attack by subdividing the problem into manageable components. Some idea of what these were can be deduced from looking at a few of the projects funded under the first ACS research budget in 1946: "The Mechanism of Protein Synthesis," "Virus Infection as a Cause of Cancer," The Effect of Caloric Restriction on Cancer Formation," and "Study of Metastatic Lesions by Means of Radioactive Tracers."

However, after some ten years, criticism of the NRC's review system forced the Society to institute its own committees of experts as peer reviewers of grant proposals. The research program has since been greatly expanded—it now includes grants to institutions for large-scale, multi-disciplinary projects; postdoctoral fellowships; physician research-training fellowships; lifetime research and clinical research professorships; special long-term institutional grants into the environmental causes of cancer; and many others.

Today, the ACS receives about 2,500 applications for research support annually. About 1,500 are specific proposals. All are judged and rated at four levels of review.

The process starts with eleven Scientific Advisory Committees, each composed of eighteen to twenty volunteer scientists or physicians, all recognized authorities. These committees are built around such subjects as immunology and immunotherapy, cell developmental biology; prevention; diagnosis and therapy. The committees rate proposals on a scale of one to five.

As practicing investigators, committee members are able to judge whether new proposals duplicate or overlap ongoing or past research. They are aware of the training and reputations of the would-be grantees and their institutions, and understand the practicalities of the project. Hence they can decide whether a proposal is sound and original, and whether the investigator is likely to have the talent and experience to carry it to conclusion within the budget he/she proposes.

The second level of review is the ACS Research Council, composed of twenty-two of volunteer senior scientists. They examine the rankings given to proposals by the Scientific Advisory Committees, including projects that have been turned down, and sometimes ask for re-review. The Council decides the cutoff level at which grants rated by the Advisory Committees will be funded.

The third level of ACS review is the Research and Clinical Investigation Committee of the Board of Directors, made up not only of senior researchers but well-informed lay people.

Finally, the rated projects go to the full ACS Board of Directors. No ACS staff person has a vote at any level of the research review process.

Currently, the ACS annual research budget is about seventy million dollars; since the inception of the Society's research program in 1945, it has invested nearly nine hundred million dollars in research, nearly one-third of its total budget.

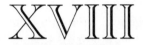

Research:
The End of Cancer

On November 17, 1982, Dr. J. Michael Bishop of the University of California, San Francisco, told the Lasker Award Luncheon guests in New York City:

> After centuries of bewilderment, the human intellect has finally laid hold of cancer with a grip that may eventually extract the deadly secrets of the disease. . . . We owe the strength of our newfound grip to the study of tumor viruses. . . . [They] have been found in human cancer. And tumor viruses have revealed to us a set of human genes whose activities may lie at the very heart of every cancer, no matter what its cause. The enemy has been found—it is part of us—and we have begun to understand the lines of its attack.

The Lasker Awards, which often anticipate Nobel Prizes (forty-two previous Lasker winners have become Nobel laureates) were given to six people in 1982 for breakthroughs in viral research, and for the discovery through virology that certain genes can cause human cancer.

Dr. Hidesaburo Hanafusa of Rockefeller University had demonstrated how a group of viruses called "retroviruses" (unlike normal viruses, which replicate DNA, they replicate messenger RNA) capture animal genes. When these viruses are reintroduced into the same animals (including humans), they cause cancers. Dr. Bishop and a colleague, Dr. Harold E. Varmus, who is an ACS lifetime research professor, shared a Lasker Award for showing that these cancer genes, known as onc genes, or oncogenes, are found in noncancerous, normal cells. They are not new genes—they are found in ancient species, indicating that they play a needed role in normal cells. But under some circumstances they are able to create cancer. Dr. Raymond L. Erikson of Harvard University, an ACS lifetime research professor who was another Lasker Award winner, had identified an enzyme produced by one of the onc genes that altered cellular metabolism. And Dr. Robert C. Gallo of the National Cancer Institute was honored by the Lasker Foundation for two important discoveries:

One: He located the place on a human chromosome where an onc gene could be found.

Two: He discovered the first human retrovirus. (A number of retroviruses had been found to cause cancer in animals since the first such virus was discovered in chicken sarcoma in 1911 by the late Dr. Peyton Rous.) Dr. Gallo's retrovirus is known as Human Thymus-Cell Leukemia Virus—or HTLV. It causes a form of leukemia that affects T cells, which are a vital part of the body's immune system. This kind of leukemia is rare in the United States but common in some parts of Japan.

In 1983, as a result of these and other findings, there was a sudden surge of optimism among cancer experts. Venturing even further into hopeful prediction than Dr. Bishop, reputable scientists began to say that the core understanding of how the disease begins was at hand. After nearly a half-century of expanded research, science appeared to be closing in on the molecular events that change a normal cell into a cancerous one. Besides the discoveries honored by the 1982 Lasker Awards, basic science had revealed important new possibilities of diagnosing and treating cancer. One was "monoclonal antibodies"—specific antibodies that can seek out and attack cancer cells, or carry radioactive charges or anticancer drugs directly to tumors without harming healthy tissue. The other finding was the anticancer properties of "interferons," one group of natural substances known as biological modifiers that are secreted by the body in response to viral infections.

Based on these synergistic advances, the leading British science journal *Nature* boldly stated that "carcinogenesis [may be] finally understood. For the first time there is a chance of getting to the bottom of the phenomenon of cancer." And Dr. Lewis Thomas, chancellor of Memorial Sloan-Kettering Cancer Center in New York City, said that the end of cancer could come "before this century is over." In fact, he wrote, "I now believe it could begin to fall into place at almost any time, starting next year or even next week. . . ." Dr. Vincent T. DeVita, director of the National Cancer Institute, said it was possible that "by the year 2000 we may not have cancer. . . . The speed of advance has been enormous."

And Dr. Frank R. Rauscher, former director of NCI and currently senior vice-president for research at the American Cancer Society, noted, "This is one of those very rare times in the history of biology in which we seem ready to make a quantum leap."

As Dr. Bishop indicated, several of these breakthroughs merge into new understanding of the carcinogenic process; it is not possible to say which is most important. The American Cancer Society has supported and continues to support research seeking to exploit all of these openings.

Oncogenes

In various estimates the human body contains between 60 trillion (60,000,000,000,000) to more than 100 quadrillion (100,000,000,000,000,000) cells. Every human cell contains perhaps 100,000 genes—each carrying a specific message. The message is delivered sometimes as an enzyme, sometimes as a structure. Each cell contains the genetic information needed to replicate the entire body, but only certain genes are switched on at any moment.

Genes are arranged on H-shaped chromosomes. There are forty-six chromosomes in every cell, each containing more than six feet of tightly coiled DNA. DNA encodes the genetic information of the cell, the purpose the cell is meant to fulfill. When the cell divides, its DNA must be replicated precisely, with its genes in the proper sequence, or the daughter cells will not perform functions identical to those of the mother cell.

DNA (and RNA, the substance that carries the message enabling cells to transcribe DNA when they divide) is made up of strands of four chemical compounds in various sequences. Each sequence is the genetic message, in code.

Cells of a certain human cancer known as Burkitt's lymphoma, largely found among African children, contain abnormal chromosomes. Burkitt's lymphoma is a cancer of B cells (bone-marrow cells), the other type of immune cell. The abnormal chromosomes of Burkitt's lymphoma cells carry a misplaced gene known as a *myc* gene, which has somehow moved from its normal location to another part of the chromosome where antibody molecules are coded. The *myc* gene is not of itself carcinogenic; it acquires its ability to create cancer when it is picked up by a retrovirus and reintroduced into normal cells.

This is how Dr. Bishop describes one possible scenario for the initiation of cancer:

> In cells DNA is transcribed into a strand of messenger RNA and the RNA is translated into protein. An infecting virus insinuates its genetic information [viruses, too, carry genes, but they have many fewer genes than do cells] into the cellular machinery, so that the cell synthesizes viral proteins specified by viral genes. The proteins synthesize many copies of the viral genome [a genome is the totality of genetic information in the cell], construct new virus particles and execute any other instructions of the viral genes. In some instances the instructions include a command that converts the host cell to a cancerous state.

Researchers Robert A. Weinberg of MIT (a longtime ACS grantee) and Geoffrey Cooper of Harvard Medical

School have isolated genes from the DNA of tumors that were *not* induced by viruses or retroviruses but which can turn normal laboratory cells into cancer cells. Known as protogenes, they are not the same as those found in retroviruses but are normal cellular genes that can be made to produce cancers. Different normal genes are found in different types of cancer; although the same gene has been found in Burkitt's lymphoma, several leukemias, neuroiblastoma, carcinoma of the colon, and two sarcomas—totally different types of tumors.

It has been discovered that parts of a chromosome can break off at weak points in its structure and exchange places with pieces of another chromosome. This phenomenon, known as translocation, creates abnormal chromosomes. Certain genes—perhaps only forty or fifty of the thousands in human cells—are positioned at these chromosomal breaks. These are growth-regulating genes, and they behave normally in their ordained places, but when moved to unaccustomed places, however, they may be switched on to produce cells that lack the self-regulating characteristic of normal cells and thus grow without cease until they form tumors.

It is not known what causes these phenomena, but their existence demonstrates how a good many cancers get started, something that had not previously been known. It is speculated that translocations may be caused by a virus or a carcinogenic chemical.

Oncogenes are the same as normal genes, and those that cause cancer in the cell do not seem to be different from the normal mechanisms of the cell. This is "unnerving," Dr. Bishop wrote in 1982. "This suggests that the design of rational therapeutic strategies [against cancer] may remain almost as vexing as it is today."

However, the speed of discovery is accelerating in oncogene research. New facets are constantly being uncovered. It is entirely possible that oncogenes may not only explain cancer but may be exploited to prevent or treat it.

Monoclonal Antibodies

The discoveries of oncogenes were made possible by a series of technical advances during the 1970s in molecular biology, most specifically the technique known as gene splicing. Scientists learned to detect a single protein among thousands, to isolate a single gene, and to sever discrete fragments of DNA and insert single genes into strands of DNA.

Two scientists working at the MRC Laboratories of Molecular Biology in Cambridge, England, made another discovery with an enormous variety of implications and applications, although they did not realize it at the time. In 1975 George Kohler and Cesar Milstein were working on antibody molecules. (An antibody is a protein created by the body's immune system to fight an antigen—which may be a bacterium, or a poison, or some other substance foreign to the body. They were interested in finding out whether parts of different antibodies could be combined to make synthetic antibodies. Wrote J. L. Fox in an article in *Chemical & Engineering News*:

> To answer that question, Milstein and Kohler tried fusing different cell types, which by themselves made distinguishable antibodies. For various reasons—partly just because certain of these cell types were conveniently available—Milstein and Kohler fused mouse spleen [a source of antibodies] with mouse myeloma cells, a kind of tumor cell that produces antibodies of unpredictable specificity.
> "The experiments were incredibly successful," Milstein recalls. "Only later did we realize the potential of the procedure. It could be done to make any antibody. And it's no longer a mixture, but a well-defined chemical."

Through various technical steps, Kohler and Milstein were able to do something that had never before been accomplished: They fused a cell capable of producing an antibody—

a spleen cell—with a cancer cell, which is immortal. The resulting hybrid cell, known as a hybridoma, had the ideal qualities of both its parents: It could produce antibodies and, unlike normal spleen cells, which are almost impossible to cultivate, it was not only easy to grow but never died. Replicating hybridomas could produce a single antibody in what to a scientist are huge quantities.

Until the hybridoma, the only way to produce antibodies was by injecting an animal with an antigen and harvesting the serum. It was in this way that various antisera were produced for immunization. However, they weren't made up of a single antibody, they were heteregenous mixes of all of the animal's antibodies. Now it is possible to culture only the antibody that is wanted. Being able to create quantities of specific antibodies opens enormous possibilities in the diagnosis and treatment of cancer, as well as a host of other prospects, including very sensitive and accurate diagnostic tests of various pathologies.

Several cancer patients have been successfully treated with the new antibodies, made specifically for their tumors. The first to be reported in 1982, was a sixty-seven-year-old man at Stanford University Medical Center in Palo Alto, California. He had been suffering from B-cell lymphoma, a rare cancer of the lymphatic system. Despite two years of treatment with chemotherapy and interferon, the disease had spread to the man's liver, spleen, bone marrow, and blood. He was in intense pain.

Dr. Ronald Levy and associates were able to culture antibodies from the man's blood and make hybridoma cells that cloned a large supply of these (monoclonal) antibodies. The process took six months. Then the antibody was injected into the patient. Within three weeks the patient's enlarged lymph nodes shrank, the liver and spleen were reduced to normal proportions, and other tumors disappeared. A year and a half later, the man was still disease-free.

The time and cost of producing antibodies for each

patient militate against making the monoclonal antibodies for treatment. Besides, using antibodies as therapy didn't work well in other of Dr. Levy's patients who had other kinds of tumors. But these proteins offer other, more wide-ranging possibilities. Since they can be made specific for various tumors, they can be used for diagnosis, and for other types of therapy. Here's how:

- The antibody can be fused with a radioactive isotope with a short half-life. When the antibody has sought out the tumor(s), a scanning device could spot and measure radioactivity to determine the size and location of the tumor(s).
- When this has been determined, doctors can decide on therapy. If they wish to use radiation, more powerful, longer-lived radioactive substances could be attached to the antibody to carry a destructive charge directly into the tumor.
- Or, if the doctors decide on chemotherapy, they could use the most poisonous drugs. Attached to antibodies, these would be taken directly to tumor cells. Thus chemotherapy, which has been hazardous because anti-cancer drugs are poisonous and do not discriminate very carefully between healthy and cancer cells, could be targeted only to cancer cells, and normal cells would be spared. The effect has been likened to a rifle or a laser, as opposed to a shotgun.

INTERFERON

"We try to use our research funds not merely as a second source to scientists, but to seek voids and opportunities in national research programs and fill them," said Dr. Frank R. Rauscher, ACS senior vice president for research, recently. "Interferons are a good example. The American Cancer Society was able to commit two million dollars to interferon cancer research in five weeks. It would take the National Cancer Institute about eighteen months to get a project like that under way—not because the NCI is slow, but because it's hampered to some extent by bureaucratic requirements."

Discovered in 1957, interferon is a natural body substance that is secreted to fight viral infections. It is species-specific—that is, the interferon made by one species of animal is effective only in that species. In the 1960s an American researcher working in France, Dr. Ian Gresser, decided to test mouse interferon against mouse leukemia, in a special strain of mouse prone to that disease. He found that the substance was not only antiviral, but antimitotic. That is, animals which would ordinarily have developed leukemia did not do so, and leukemic mice lived longer when treated with interferon.

Other researchers had similar experience with interferon in chickens, hamsters, and other species. But there was no interferon made for use in human disease until Dr. K. Cantell of the Finnish national blood bank began producing the substance in the mid 1970s. Stockholm's Karolinska Institute was the first to test it in patients. The compound was given to twenty-eight patients with osteogenic sarcoma, a bone cancer, after treatment with radiation and/or surgery. A modest increase in survival was demonstrated in these patients.

Others were able to buy small quantities of interferon from Finland, but it was prohibitively expensive. Enough of the substance to treat a single cancer patient costs about $50,000.

The few who received interferon seemed to do better than expected. But this is what investigators call "anecdotal evidence." A means of following blood levels of interferon in patients was developed, and the possibility of clinical research expanded. Leading investigators Drs. Jordan Gutterman of M. D. Anderson Hospital in Houston, Texas and Thomas Merigan of Stanford University went to Dr. Rauscher, then head of the National Cancer Institute, and asked him to put up $5 million to buy enough interferon for clinical experimentation.

Dr. Rauscher sent a team to Sweden to study the results at Karolinska. They returned urging caution: The trials had used "historical controls"—that is, results in present patients given interferon were compared with those treated years earlier without it. There are three types of osteogenic sarcoma. One is much less virulent, but the Swedish trials had not separated them.

Instead of buying $5 million worth of interferon, Dr. Rauscher committed a half-million dollars to an attempt to sequence its proteins to make a synthetic, inexpensive version that would be available in quantity. This chemical analysis had not succeeded when Dr. Rauscher left the NCI and moved to the American Cancer Society in 1976. A year or so later, he began to get more calls about interferon from Gutterman, Merigan, and other investigators. They were reporting increasingly intriguing results, and they wanted to be able to buy enough interferon to do comparative studies.

Rauscher was now convinced. He went to Lane Adams and said, "I think we ought to bite this bullet." It was not the first time that Adams had heard of interferon. Dr. Gutterman had been keeping Mary Lasker informed of his progress against breast cancer with the compound, and she had passed this on to Adams.

Adams agreed that something ought to be done. An ad hoc committee of national directors was created, and Dr. Rauscher told them he wanted $2 million to buy interferon from Finland. It was by far the largest amount ever asked for a single project by the ACS. But it was voted and committed.

"I called Cantell and told him we needed fifty billion units of interferon," Dr. Rasucher recalled recently.

The ACS wanted to answer several basic questions: Was interferon active against cancer patients? What tumors? What was the dosage, when should it be given, when should it be stopped? And there was a third goal: by committing so much money, the ACS hoped to induce the federal government and private industry to become involved in making more interferon. When the ACS committed its first $2 million (the total is now close to $8 million), there was only enough interferon in the world to treat 150 cancer patients, and, of course, it was extremely expensive.

Soon after the ACS announced its support of the interferon program, the Shell Oil Company Foundation told Dr. Rauscher they were interested in making a grant. Out of this came a $1 million donation to ACS, earmarked for interferon.

Impressed by the heavy ACS involvement, a number of large pharmaceutical and genetic engineering companies began to study and try to produce interferon. Several have succeeded.

The questions about its effectiveness against cancer, have now been partially answered. There are six tumors in which interferon is effective. Five of these are cancer: hairy-cell leukemia (dramatic response); chronic myeloid leukemia; Kaposi's sarcoma; non-Hodgkin's lymphoma; kidney cancer (produces response, even after metastasis); and bladder cancer. The sixth tumor is not malignant, but a very dangerous disease: larynegeal papilomas (warts).

A great deal has been learned about interferon. At least fourteen different types have been identified. They seem to vary in effectiveness depending on the tumor they are used to treat. Moreover, huge amounts of interferon are now available. Twelve different genes have been captured that can make interferon, and many of the major gene-splicing companies such as Genentech and Biogen are making it as well as many large pharmaceutical firms: Hoffmann-LaRoche, Schering Plough, Burroughs Wellcome. These interferons are pure, simplifying treatment and permitting a clearer evaluation, whereas early Finnish interferon was a mix of about .1 percent of interferon with many other substances.

Where 6 million units were given daily per patient in 1979, today the daily dose may be as high as one hundred and fifty million units. And the cost of interferon for a full course of treatments has plummeted.

HUMAN CANCER VIRUS

Interferons seem to work mainly by stimulating the body's natural immune defenses to create killer cells that attack cancer cells—and perhaps by other immunological pathways as well.

Sponsoring interferon research into Kaposi's sarcoma, the Society became the first agency to investigate ways of controlling the new scourge known as acquired immune deficiency syndrome (AIDS.) Kaposi's sarcoma, a tenacious tumor, is one of the rarer causes of death from the dreaded, and so far incurable, AIDS. However, any advance against AIDS is noteworthy. In clinical trials at Memorial Sloan-Kettering Hospital in New York City, the type of interferon known as alpha-interferon has had a remarkably high temporary response rate in patients with Kaposi's sarcoma.

"Research we funded on both coasts in 1980 prompted a great deal of interest in AIDS," Dr. Rauscher remarked recently. "It got the whole field moving much earlier than it otherwise might have."

Interferon's effectiveness encouraged research into other, similar biological modifiers. Dr. Robert C. Gallo of the National Cancer Institute began investigating T(hymus) cells, white cells that circulate through the body as part of the immune system. T cells were thought to be the targets of virus particles, which created certain rare forms of leukemia as well as AIDS. But it was impossible to grow T cells in the laboratory, and without them there was no way to extract the virus.

Dr. Gallo isolated an enzyme, known as a lymphokine, that stimulated the growth of T cells. He called it T cell growth factor; it's now known as Interleuken 2 or IL2. Using this substance, Dr. Gallo was able to grow enough T cells to prospect for the suspected virus. And in this way, he was able to achieve one of the greatest breakthroughs in cancer research. He found the first human cancer virus, human T cell leukemia virus, or HTLV I. Dr. Gallo has since shown that HTLV I is widely prevalent in certain areas of the world: the Caribbean, Central and South America, parts of Africa, and the southeastern United States. It is not highly infectious.

Dr. Gallo has found two other viruses in the same family—HTLV II and III. One of these is of enormous importance. HTLV III has been proved to be the cause of AIDS. The virus is now being used in diagnostic tests that can determine whether blood samples are safe for transfusion. And there is hope that a vaccine against AIDS may be developed from this deadly virus.

IL2 has since been shown to have remarkable properties beyond the ability to stimulate growth of T cells. It appears to increase their immune properties as well—and perhaps have a generalized immune effect against cancer. As a result, Dr. Steven A. Rosenberg of NCI and his research team have been using IL2 in a technique known as "adoptive immunity."

It works this way: White cells are removed from cancer patients and cultured with IL2. These immunologically strengthened cells are then reinfused into the patients along with an additional dose of IL2. In some twenty-five patients with a variety of far advanced cancers (i.e., not expected to survive), this technique has shown early, promising results. But Dr. Rosenberg strongly urges caution: The treatment is in its earliest experimental stage, and is no magic cure for cancer.

OTHER BIOLOGICAL MODIFIERS

Encouraged by the work in interferon and IL2, other ACS-supported researchers are exploring other biological modifiers, some of which are becoming available in quantity from manufacturers:

- Tumor Necrosis Factor (TNF): a tumor-killing protein made by white blood cells that is potentially effective against a broad range of cancers. It can also stimulate the release of one type of interferon (gamma).
- Colony-Stimulating Factor (CSF): A group of proteins that stimulate macrophages—large scavenger cells—that dispose of foreign substances in the body. Macrophages can also attack and kill tumor cells.
- Cytlysin and Leukoreglin: recently discovered products of the immune system, which appear to affect the immune stimulating power of IL2, and to block the proliferation of tumor cells. Not yet extracted in pure form, they have therefore not yet been produced in quantity for experimentation.

CHEMOPREVENTION

The connection between what we eat—or don't—and cancer has fascinated physicians, scientists, and the public for many years; during the past couple of decades, this broad question has been focused into specific research.

A substantial body of studies began to suggest that a number of compounds, known to be safe for human beings *in small quantities*, as well as certain foods, may help prevent human cancer or the spread of cancer.

Starting in 1982, the National Cancer Institute and the American Cancer Society began larger research programs into the cancer-control properties of certain vitamins, vegetables and fruits, and minerals. This field is known as chemoprevention—a newly coined word. It means preventing cancer with chemical means (the definition of *chemical* is a broad one) or turning it off after it starts.

The chemopreventive substances under study are:

- Vitamins A, C and E;
- Beta-carotene, the coloring compound in carrots and

yellow fruits and vegetables, which is a "precursor" of vitamin A, i.e., the body forms vitamin A from it:

- Retinoids, substances that are synthetic chemical cousins of vitamin A, and hopefully less toxic than that substance;
- Selenium, a sulfurlike element;
- A food additive known as BHA;
- Certain beans, such as soy and kidney beans;
- Brussels sprouts, cabbage, broccoli;
- Green coffee beans;
- Black tea.

Experimental evidence indicates that these substances work against cancer in different ways, not all of which are wholly understood.

Vitamin A and retinoids: Vitamin A seems to have an "inverse associaiton" with cancer in animals and human patients; i.e., the more vitamin A, the less cancer. The blood levels of vitamin A in male cancer patients were lower than that in healthy men, but this could be an effect of the disease, rather than a causative factor. In laboratory animals, vitamin A has been shown to protect against skin cancer and perhaps tumors caused by chemicals. It's an important component of "epithelial" cells—the cells that form skin, and line the intestines and blood vessels. About 50 percent of all cancers form in epithelial cells.

However, there are strong caveats against giving substantial amounts of vitamin A to people. Being fat soluble, vitamin A is stored in the body, mainly in the liver, and it cannot be taken by humans in doses large enough to affect cancer without first poisoning them. Science has synthesized hundreds of analogues of vitamin A—chemical cousins known as retinoids, some of which are less toxic to people than vitamin A. Perhaps one of these may be developed as a protection against cancer for human beings.

Vitamins C and E: Both these vitamins are antioxidants—

they help prevent spoilage. In fact, the major use of vitamin C is as a food preservative. Both vitamins can block nitrates, found in natural vegetables and preserved meats, from linking with amines in the body or in meats. When nitrates and amines join, they form nitrosamines, known to cause cancer. Hence, both vitamins may be protective against the formation of these carcinogens, and perhaps, others. Investigations among populations with high rates of stomach and esophageal cancer in Chile, China, Colombia, and Iran indicate that vitamin C in the diet may protect against these tumors. Animal experiments support this.

Vitamin C is water-soluble; vitamin E is fat soluble. Eating vitamin C, or adding some to frying bacon, may block nitrosamine formation; however, C lasts for only four minutes in a heated frying pan and acts only on lean meat. To prevent nitrosamine formation in cooking, the fat part of bacon requires the addition of fat soluble vitamin E, which does not disintegrate under heat.

Selenium: In rats, cancer induced by chemicals can be blocked by adding selenium to their drinking water.

Other experiments have shown that exposing bacteria to a certain chemical may cause gene changes known as mutations. A chemical that causes mutations is considered to be a probable carcinogen. Adding selenium to the laboratory dish holding the bacteria and the chemical reduces the mutagenic activity of the chemical.

Peoples' diets contain widely varying amounts of selenium, depending on what they eat and where it comes from. Seafood and organ meats are rich in selenium. High mortality rates from colon, rectal, and breast cancer in Maine have been linked with selenium-poor soil; but this is only suggestive evidence as it's common for Americans to eat foods grown in other states. China and Finland have been adding selenium to their drinking water to offset possible cancers that might result from a lack of the element in their food supplies.

BHA: BHA is a chemical additive used to preserve baked goods and to prevent rancidity in cooking oils. It has been demonstrated that this widely used compound detoxifies substances in the body known to cause cancer. In experiments, it has been fed to animals in high doses (100 milligrams per kilogram of body weight) for years without harm. It is being clinically tested for toxicity and effectiveness in human beings.

WARNING: While all of the substances discussed above are harmless to humans in tiny amounts, and almost all are easily purchased (BHA is available only in bulk to food processors), several may be poisonous in larger doses: Vitamins E and A, and selenium, are examples. There are no guidelines for dosing individuals with any of these substances at this time. While scientists investigate suggestive evidence, people are cautioned against jumping to conclusions about the efficacy of any of these substances in preventing or reversing cancer.

In 1984 the American Cancer Society issued dietary recommendations designed to lower cancer risk for Americans. These recommendations included:

- Avoiding obesity (associated with a higher rate of cancers of the uterus, gallbladder, kidney, stomach, colon and breast);
- Lowering fat intake (high-fat diets are associated with greater risk of cancers of the breast, colon, and prostate);
- Eating more fiber-rich grain cereals, fruits, and vegetables, at least as a substitute for fatty foods;
- Including dark-green leafy or yellow vegetables and fruits in the diet (for vitamins C and A, and carotene);
- Including vegetables of the cabbage family in the diet (may protect against gastrointestinal and respiratory cancers);

- Moderating intake of alcoholic beverages (large alcohol intake is associated with esophageal cancer risk in France, certain African countries, and elsewhere);
- Moderating consumption of salt-cured, smoked, and nitrite-cured foods (real smoke may leave carcinogenic tar residue). There is inferential evidence from China and Scandinavia that heavy consumption of salt-cured, pickled, and nitrite-cured foods may be linked with stomach and esophageal cancers.

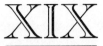

XIX

Clinical Research: To Help the Cancer Patient

Dr. C. Gordon Zubrod, director of the Comprehensive Cancer Center of the State of Florida, in Miami, estimates that almost all cures of cancer have taken place since about 1880, and that the rate of cure has gone up about 1 percent every two and a half years "and there is evidence that the pace quickens."

The source of progress is mainly research—first basic research of the kind already discussed, and then clinical research in patients with cancer.

In 1970 a panel of experts on the conquest of cancer defined

Clinical investigation [as] essentially the culmination of basic and preclinical studies in cancer research and the development from these of techniques useful in preventing, diagnosing, and treating cancer in man. Among the important achievements of clinical investigation have been the testing of new surgical procedures, new types of ionizing radiation, and new chemotherapeutic agents in man and the devleopment of schedules and combinations of therapies that have resulted in great improvement in treatment. For certain types of cancer, cures or presumed cures ("presumed" because insufficient time has elapsed) have been achieved by chemotherapy in patients with choriocarcinomas and Burkitt's tumor and occasionally in patients with widespread Hodgkin's disease, acute leukemia and other forms of cancer for which the previous cure rate was virtually zero.

143

Since 1970, those presumed cures have become actual cures, and others have been added to the list.

There has always been a debate, sometimes rancorous, about where money for cancer research ought to go. Some scientists feel that basic research is scanted when money is put into clinical trials. To clinicians, the patient must be primary—all of their training is aimed at helping the man, woman, or child who has cancer. In fact, both basic and clinical research are needed, and the best minds in both areas are constantly weighing alternatives and priorities in an attempt to keep an intelligent balance in funding. The ideal of cancer control is joining both types of research "to close the gap between what we know and what we do," as Dr. John R. Heller once put it.

The late Congressman Daniel Flood of Pennsylvania, former head of the House of Representatives subcommittee that supervised funds for cancer research, once spelled this out:

> I have a right to expect and I think I'm in a position to demand that you keep the patient foremost—not the lab, nor the department, nor the academic journal [all those are necessary] but the patient foremost in mind. . . . Serendipity [the chance discovery of useful information] is a *sine qua non* of basic research. But we can no longer leave to serendipity the wending of a research product from the laboratory to the patient.

Because clinical investigations try new methods in patients, the charge is frequently made that the patients are treated as guinea pigs. Replying to one such criticism by two Washington reporters, Dr. Vincent T. DeVita, an oncologist honored for several major advances in chemotherapy of cancer, and head of the National Cancer Institute, wrote in 1981:

> Cancer patients—and the doctors treating them—have as their first goal the successful treatment of the disease. . . . Cancer is lethal if left untreated. The possibility of treatment side effects

and the small but real chance of drug-related death has to be balanced against the nearly 100 percent chance of death if experimental therapy is not attempted for the advanced cancer patients who participate in our studies.

Clinical investigation is often stimulated by the observations of trained clinicians and epidemiologists.

The theory of cancer until the late nineteenth century was that solid tumors were at first always localized. Hence, the only widely accepted treatment was surgical removal. When ionizing radiation was discovered by Roentgen in 1895, that, too, was applied to cancers, but it could not affect underlying tumors without severely damaging skin and intervening healthy tissue.

In the 1890s, clinical observation led to a new theory about malignant growth. It began to be believed that even early tumors sometimes spread cancer cells to regional lymph nodes, and a new type of radical surgery was developed to deal with this—the Halsted radical mastectomy is the best-known example. If patients weren't cured, it was deemed that surgery had been insufficient, so increasingly radical operations were devised.

"However, even when the surgeon and the radiation oncologist have done their best in patients who seem to have localized/regional disease, many patients die of metastatic cancer," wrote Dr. Zubrod. He calculated in 1980 that treating the tumors with even the most radical surgery would fail in 86 percent of lung-cancer cases, 60 percent of stomach cancers, 47 percent of colorectal cases, and 33 percent of breast cancers. "This failure rate is a rough approximation of the degree to which cancer was not a localized/regional disease at the time of diagnosis," Zubrod wrote. "The flaw in this concept of regional containment began to be recognized in the mid-1950s when tumor cells were demonstrated in the circulating blood."

From then on, the concept began to change. Even

though cancer seemed confined to a tumor, it was increasingly accepted that "micrometastases" probably existed in distant organs. Something was needed to wipe out those invisible colonies.

There was a time, not long ago, when the great majority of physicians thought that the only proper use for drugs in cancer was to relieve pain. The concept of using medications to treat the disease seemed chimerical—there was so little difference between normal cells and cancer cells. One researcher said it was like trying to find a substance that, taken internally, would dissolve the right ear while leaving the left ear untouched.

It was true, according to Dr. Zubrod, that "drugs that could cause remission of clinical cancer have been known for at least two millennia." But truly effective and reasonably safe medications were not found until the 1940s. Discovered to be highly active in animal cancers, nitrogen mustard, the antifolics, and cortisone proved most effective against certain widely disseminated cancers in human beings: the leukemias and lymphomas.

Since these early cancer drugs worked, they demonstrated empirically that there were differences between cancer cells and normal cells. Thus, new drugs continued to be developed under a major program of the National Cancer Institute and by private pharmaceutical companies. The ACS also funded research in this field. One of the most potent cancer drug discoveries—5-fluorouracil—came from Dr. Charles Heidelberger, an American Cancer Society research professor. Today there are more than fifty drugs useful against human cancer, and they are the treatment of choice in at least a dozen forms of the disease. They are curing formerly incurable cancers, and are even sometimes effective against advanced, widely disseminated disease.

Dr. Joseph H. Burchenal of Memorial Sloan-Kettering Hospital in New York put it neatly: "Surgery and radiotherapy are limited not only by the bulk of the tumor, but by its dissemination, whereas . . . chemotherapy is limited by the mass of the tumor, rather than its dissemination." Surgery and radiation are essentially restricted to removing or destroying solid tumors, whereas drugs can hit cancer cells anywhere in the body but are relatively ineffective against large solid tumors. Thus, it made sense to join the three modalities in treating patients.

After surgery some specialists began administering anti-cancer drugs. The best example is in breast cancer, where surgery is used to remove the tumor, and "adjuvant ther-apy"—various courses and combinations of chemotherapy—is administered to kill any other cancer cells that may exist in the body. The first such adjuvant treatment combination was developed against breast cancer in the 1950s by Dr. Bernard Fisher and colleagues of the NCI. A ten-year follow-up in 1968 showed slightly better survival among patients who were given three days of thiotepa—an anticancer drug—after breast surgery.

Later, more drugs were used in treating breast cancer in a longer postsurgery course, and surgery no longer automati-cally meant the Halsted radical mastectomy, or the modified radical mastectomy, or even the simple mastectomy. Lum-pectomy (tumor removal) followed by radiation therapy be-came a standard treatment in appropriate cases. And in some breast cancers radiotherapy without surgery was the major treatment modality. Therapy was considerably less mutilat-ing, and five- and ten-year survival improved. Both of these changes have encouraged women with breast lumps to come to their doctors earlier, thus improving their chances—and the overall statistics—of survival.

One of the best examples of the effectiveness of clinical research is Hodgkin's disease, named after the British doctor who first described it in 1832. This cancer invades the lymph nodes, one of the body's defenses, where infections and cancer cells are trapped. There are several hundred of these nodes throughout the body.

Medical textbooks described Hodgkin's disease as "incurable" well into the 1960s. Then in 1963 the late Dr. Eric C. Easson, director of the Christie Hospital and Holt Radium Institute in Manchester, England, published an article in the *British Medical Journal* with the daring title "The Cure of Hodgkin's Disease." The medical profession was, of course, skeptical if not totally disbelieving, but Dr. Easson could prove what he was talking about with his own and other clinical studies.

Soon after the discovery of ionizing radiation, some adventurous radiologists had turned their primitive machines on Hodgkin's disease. This equipment put out long waves that burned the skin before they could reach underlying tumors. And harmful rays scattered uncontrollably. A handful of patients were helped, but many were harmed.

In the 1920s, Dr. René Gilbert, a Swiss radiologist, began experimenting with the then higher-voltage X-ray machines. Using special filters to direct the rays more precisely, Dr. Gilbert was able to destroy some Hodgkin's tumors, and to keep the disease at bay when it recurred. In 1939 he reported a 35-percent five-year survival rate among fifty-four patients.

Doctors were still skeptical that Hodgkin's disease could be controlled. But a Toronto radiologist, Dr. Gordon E. Richards, tried Gilbert's methods and achieved similar results. Dr. Vera Peters, trained by Dr. Richards at the Ontario Institute of Radiotherapy, carried his work forward and began attacking the disease ever more aggressively. One of her first patients, around 1935, was a twenty-eight-year-old laborer who "presented" with the most frequent first symptom of the disease, a painless tumor in the left side of his neck. He also had a swollen node under his left arm.

Dr. Peters gave him a heavy dose (3,000 rads) of radiation over a four-week period, and the tumors disappeared. Five years later his disease recurred in the abdomen. Further radiation again wiped it out. In fact, the man was treated for recurrences for twenty years, during which time nearly every lymph node in his body was irradiated. After 1952 he had no further recurrences.

Dr. Peters developed a technique for giving lighter, "precautionary" doses of radiation to nodes near the site of cancer. In 1950 she reported on 113 Hodgkin's disease patients treated between 1928 and 1942: Fifty-one percent survived for five years, and 35 percent were still living ten years after treatment, a large number of them free of disease.

At that time Dr. Peters concluded that the chief factors in controlling Hodgkin's disease were early diagnosis and a more optimistic attitude about prognosis: If doctors believed a patient with Hodgkin's disease was incurable, they would do nothing to add to his discomfort. They would, therefore, avoid giving high levels of radiation, which may cause nausea and other disagreeable effects.

Dr. Peters's clinical investigations spurred Dr. Henry S. Kaplan—late ACS president and professor of radiology at Stanford Univeristy Medical Center, Palo Alto, California—to carry forward the attack on Hodgkin's lymphoma. Dr. Peters had done her work with kilovoltage equipment, which generated only about 250,000 volts of radiation. During World War II, however, industry had needed more powerful radiation to inspect parts of weapons and machines for flaws. An apparatus called the "linear accelerator" was developed that emitted much more powerful, multimillion-volt, short X-rays to deeply penetrate metals and other materials. Dr. Kaplan called on Stanford's microwave electronics engineers to build a machine of this type for treating patients. Theoretically it would be able to penetrate deeply into the body while sparing the skin, and its rays would not scatter; thus malignancies adjacent to normal structures might be irradiated without harming the patient.

It took several years to raise the money to produce a unique machine with a six-foot-long vacuum tube that could shoot a 5-million-volt, rifle-sharp beam of penetrating X rays.

The first patient treated with the new linear accelerator in 1957 was a forty-one-year-old woman with stage II Hodgkin's disease: she had tumors in her neck and in the region behind the breastbone known as the mediastinum. Dr. Kaplan hit both areas with a maximum dose of 3,000 rads. The tumors disappeared and the woman remained free of cancer.

However, in similar cases the disease recurred in about 10 percent of patients. Kaplan increased the dose to a daring 4,000 rads—previously thought too large to be bearable—and the recurrence rate dropped to 1 percent.

Kaplan and other radiotherapists were still flying blind; they had no way of knowing where the disease would spread. Then, in 1962, a British surgeon invented the "lymphangio-gram," a means of outlining and making X-ray pictures of the body's lumph nodes. This gave the radiologists road maps to guide treatment.

Until then, advanced (stage III) Hodgkin's patients had been considered incurable. They had been given light radia-tion doses of 1,500 rads to relieve pain and severe itching; such doses permitted one or two supplementary radiation treatments. But perhaps these people could be cured by a risky, go-for-broke therapy that would leave no margin for future palliation.

The way to find out was through clinical experimenta-tion. Patients were divided into two groups: One got the usual low dose of X rays, the other 4,000 rads to every lymph node in the trunk and neck. Such massive radiation had never before been given so widely. It would strike most of the body's bone marrow, the main blood-forming tissue, and might cause leukemia, or make the patient vulnerable to fatal infection.

The heavy radiation dose did indeed create some cases of anemia, and opened the way to infections—although nothing as severe as anticipated. More important, the long-term sur-vival of these heavily irradiated patients was greater than that of the control group. This has become the standard treatment for many patients with advanced Hodgkin's disease.

The cure rate of early (Stage I and II) disease rose to more than 80 percent. And for patients with advanced disease, two doctors at the National Cancer Institute, Paul P. Carbone and Vincent T. DeVita, developed a combination drug treatment that proved effective and has since evolved into even more-potent therapy. Today, as many as 85 percent of patients with advanced Hodgkin's disease are being cured with one or another form of treatment developed through years of clinical investigation.

According to Dr. Saul A. Rosenberg, professor of medicine and radiology at Stanford University, "The understanding and management of patients with malignant lymphomas has been a major advance of medicine of the last 10–20 years. These advances have transformed Hodgkin's disease from a predominantly fatal illness to a curable one for the great majority of patients diagnosed in 1980."

Most of the cancers cured by chemotherapy occur in children or young adults and are characterized by a rapid proliferation of fast-growing cells. It has been shown that cells most vulnerable to drug treatments are those in some stage of mitotic division; quiescent or non-dividing cells seem able to hide from drugs. This is one of the limiting factors in cancer chemotherapy. Another is that human cancer cells sensitive to a given drug *in vitro* (in a laboratory dish) do not always respond as well to the same drug in the patient's body.

Still, effective anticancer drugs have now completely reversed the prognosis of a number of tumors. The latest is testicular cancer in young men—formerly fatal in 80 percent of cases, now about 80 percent of patients achieve a five year survival with new drugs made from platinum.

Overall, in about twenty less common forms of cancer, the cure rate with chemotherapy is 80 percent, and in breast cancer—drugs have increased the survival rate dramatically.

Altogether, about 50,000 of the 350,000 cancer patients being cured this year in the United States will be cured by chemotherapy; another 100,000 or so will be cured by radiotherapy alone or in combination with surgery; and the remainder by surgery. Furthermore, radiotherapy is being made more effective by drugs that increase tumors' uptake of oxygen and thereby make them more radiosensitive. And surgical cures are being increased with adjuvant drug therapy.

All of this is the result of scientific research translated into therapy through clinical investigations.

ACS International

Cancer knows no boundary of class, age, sex, color, religion, politics, nation, or society. It spans climates, continents, and cultures; it afflicts, indiscriminately, African bushmen and ayatollahs, commissars and congressmen.

An estimated 5,900,000 cases of cancer occurred in the world in 1975 (most recent figure). Among men, the most numerous tumors were of the lung, stomach, colon/rectum, mouth/pharynx, prostate, and esophagus, in that order. Leading sites of female cancer were breast, cervix/uterus, stomach, colon/rectum, lung, and mouth/pharynx. (When the incidences for both sexes are combined, stomach cancer is the most frequent tumor, lung is next; but the trends are toward reversal of these rankings. As cigarette smoking spreads in the third world through the high-pressure marketing of the international tobacco companies, the lung-cancer death rate is rising even among relatively young populations.) With the above sites, the leukemias and lymphomas and cancers of the liver and bladder include about 75 percent of all cancers that occurred in 1975, worldwide.

Cancer death rates vary greatly among countries. For example, the highest male cancer death rates for 1980–81 among forty-eight countries reporting such information are found in Hungary, Scotland, the Netherlands, Luxembourg, and France in that order. For women, the highest cancer death rates are in Denmark, Scotland, Luxembourg, Hungary, and Ireland. The lowest cancer death rates for men and

153

women are found in the Syrian Arab Republic. These rankings are apt to change from year to year.

Too, there are striking variations in types of tumors among different countries. Japan leads the world in male and female stomach-cancer mortality. But Japan is forty-first in deaths from breast cancer, and twenty-ninth in male lung-cancer mortality. Scotland has the highest lung-cancer death rate for men, and second highest lung-cancer death rate among the world's women, but is twenty-sixth in uterine cancer.

Dr. John Higginson, formerly of the International Agency for Research in Cancer, in Lyons, France, compared the highest and lowest frequencies of deaths from different cancers in different countries, and deduced that these variations must have been caused by "environmental factors." Many people have misunderstood Dr. Higginson's concept: They assume that he meant industrial chemical pollution of air and water. But Dr. Higginson's list of environmental factors was much broader. He included diet, smoking, drinking alcohol, and taking drugs, as well as being exposed to chemicals at work.

The American Cancer Society has based programs on reducing or avoiding known carcinogens. Those aimed at the many cancers caused by cigarette smoking are the best known. Cigarette smoking is the most widespread carcinogen identified in the environment, and its lethal effects are greater than the sum of all others known at this time. Other carcinogens are generally confined to the workplace. These include aromatic amines in the dye industry, asbestos, uranium, and chemicals used in making plastics and artificial rubber. Hepatitis B, a cause of liver cancer, is endemic in the Orient; cancer related to excessive alcohol consumption has been identified in several countries but not the United States.

Although its focus was on its own country, the American Society for the Control of Cancer early recognized the international aspects of cancer. Its managing director, Dr. George A. Soper, toured Europe in 1924, visiting the twenty-odd cancer societies that had been inspired by the success of the ASCC and looking into research and treatment facilities. He reported his findings in *Cancer Control in Europe*, which was published by the Society in 1925.

The Executive Committee decided that "the investigation of what other countries were doing in regard to cancer control had produced much useful information." This led logically to the idea of holding an international cancer symposium. The dates were September 20–24, 1926; the place Lake Mohonk, New York. "The aim is not to initiate investigations but to report upon those productive ones which have already been made."

A group of 109 cancer authorities from England, France, Germany, Denmark, and several other countries, plus many Americans, gathered at the Lake Mohonk House to discuss cancer control. They ultimately agreed on fifteen statements of "practical fact or sound working opinions . . . as the basis of the campaign which mankind should make against cancer." These said, among other things, that cancer isn't contagious or infectious; it is not hereditary; early detection is the best assurance of cure; and the public must be taught the earliest signals of cancer. Unexpectedly, the symposium generated a huge amount of press coverage, which furthered the cause of cancer control.

At a later international cancer congress in Madrid, October 1933, held under the auspices of French authorities, the delegates voted to establish a permanent International Union Against Cancer (Union Internationale Contre le Cancer, or UICC) aimed at coordinating international cancer research and control. The following year the union was established in Paris. In 1954 Mefford Runyon, the executive vice-president of the American Cancer Society, asked Miss Mildred E. Allen to find out from the UICC where other cancer societies existed. At that time the assistant secretary-general of the UICC, Dr. Pierre Denoix, sent a list of forty-eight cancer organizations.

Elmer Bobst, a leading ACS volunteer, who traveled

widely told Runyon, "We have to do something to help other countries to develop cancer societies. . . . Everywhere I went, people asked me about my work with the American Cancer Society." Mrs. Lasker was also interested in encouraging international cancer control. In 1954, at the request of Bobst and Mary Lasker, the ACS Board of Directors established a special Committee to Advance the Worldwide Fight Against Cancer "to aid and stimulate the creation of cancer societies in other countries." Dr. Alfred Popma served as its chairman for the first five years. For staff support, the ACS established a foreign desk, with Mrs. Allen—who had worked for the U.S. State Deparment—in charge. In 1966 she was joined by Gerry Schramm de Harven, who took over the foreign desk when Mrs. Allen retired in 1967. After leaving the ACS, Mildred Allen moved to Zürich, Switzerland, where she worked as a consultant to the UICC until her death in 1977.

Under Mmes. Allen and de Harven, the ACS became known as a source of help for groups in all countries who wish to establish or improve voluntary cancer societies. As the first voluntary health group to demonstrate that it is both essential and possible to involve the public in cancer control, it has provided a model for similar efforts elsewhere in the world. And as the leading voluntary health organization, the ACS has supplied information, materials, and expertise to help establish cancer societies adapted to the social, economic, and governmental structures of more than 100 countries. And it has maintained liaison with them to help forward cancer control.

Its volunteers and staff have often been invited to share their experience with other nations, including great powers whose ideologies and interests are in conflict with those of the United States and with one another, namely the Union of Soviet Socialist Republics, and the Peoples' Republic of China.

The late U.S. Senator Hubert H. Humphrey told the Senate on September 22, 1961, "It is fair to say that in my three years of study of world medical problems, I have found that no single American voluntary organization has worked more closely with voluntary health groups than has the American Cancer Society. Much of the credit for this great work goes to Mary Lasker and Elmer Bobst."

The ACS has also been a staunch supporter of the UICC, responsible for approximately one-half of that organization's budget. A number of leading ACS volunteers—including Dr. R. Lee Clark, Charles R. Ebersol, Mrs. Audrey Mars, Dr. Gerald P. Murphy, Frank Wilcox, and Armand Willig—have also worked to help make the UICC the leading organization of its kind in the world.

PART FOUR

Human Values

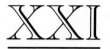

Reach to Recovery

In 1952, during my most frightening days and nights in the hospital, the outlook seemed bleakly hopeless.

Overwhelmed by anxieties so acute and so bewildering that I all but drowned in them, my mind surged with questions—some very practical but with no practical answers forthcoming, some rather foolish but nevertheless terribly serious to me, and some so highly personal I could not even bring myself to put them into words. How I ached to talk to another woman who had had the same experience and come through it, and so could counsel, and reassure, and understand!

But no such woman was available.

The woman who wrote this had just awakened from anesthesia after breast-cancer surgery at Memorial Sloan-Kettering Cancer Center in New York City. The year was 1952. She was Terese Lasser, an active, outgoing person who loved dancing and swimming, worked as a volunteer for the Red Cross, had two children, five grandchildren, and a very full life. She'd never been seriously ill, and certainly did not expect to have cancer, not even after she found a lump in her right breast. Her doctor was not worried, but thought she should see a surgeon, the famous Dr. Frank Adair, chief of the breast service at Memorial Sloan-Kettering. Dr. Adair had been reassuring—after all, the great majority of breast lumps are not cancerous. But he was also insistent: A biopsy was needed, just to be sure.

161

In 1952 the standard treatment for a suspicious breast lump was to put the patient in the hospital, anesthetize her, and surgically remove a portion of the lump. This was immediately taken to a laboratory near the operating room, where it was frozen, sliced into sections, and examined under a microscope by a pathologist. If the tissue had malignant cells, the surgeon went ahead with a mastectomy. The patient had been told, of course, that this might happen. At the time that Mrs. Lasser was treated, the Halsted procedure, which involved removing not only the affected breast but lymph nodes in the chest and under the arm as well as muscle tissue, was considered by most surgeons, especially in the United States, the form of therapy most likely to cure, the best chance of "getting it all."

Mrs. Lasser had signed the necessary consent forms, but she hadn't wanted to think about the possibility that the lump might be malignant. Like most women, she knew, or knew about, people who had had cancer—a friend's mother, a grandmother, or another relative. When these people's names were mentioned, heads were always gravely shaken.

She was fearful, yet optimistic. She couldn't believe that they would find cancer. She'd checked into the hospital expecting only the biopsy, minor surgery, not telling her husband so as not to worry him, because he'd had two heart attacks. Then she woke up after anesthesia:

> Pain lances through the numbness that is your body. To move your arm, one of your arms, is agony—but you can move the other, and you do move it. Your hand touches your side. For the first time you are aware of the bandage.
> Bandage?
> From midriff to neck, tight-wrapped as a mummy, you are bound in surgical gauze.
> Somewhere deep inside you a switch is thrown and your mind goes blank. You do not want to think, you do not want to guess, you do not want to know. But in that moment you do know.
> The impossible, the unthinkable, has happened.
> Your breast has been removed.

Dr. Adair, "a brilliant specialist and a very busy man," told her that she would have to start exercising. Exercise would counteract the aftereffects of surgery and, it was hoped, prevent edema in her arm and preserve its activity. What sort of exercise? Adair said that the nurse would teach her.

But the nurse wasn't much more helpful than the doctor: " 'Exercise of any kind,' she said, 'just so that you move your arm.' "

The advice was sound, but bewildering to a woman who had just undergone not merely drastic treatment for cancer, but major trauma to her body and psyche.

"In our bosom-oriented culture, the psychological impact of a mastectomy is unparalleled by almost any kind of surgery," wrote Dr. Arthur Holleb. "As a breast cancer surgeon, I thought I was doing a pretty good job in providing the 'pat on the back,' the reassuring 'Don't worry, my dear, everything will be like it was before,' and providing the name of a local corsetiere. . . . Little did I know!"

Mrs. Lasser was not only left to invent her own exercises, she was not even told where and how to shop for an artificial breast. She didn't know that it wasn't merely a cosmetic device but also provided weight to balance her other breast. She wasn't informed that it was called a prosthesis. More important, there was no one to answer her questions about herself. The underlying and overriding fear for most women who have mastectomies is whether their husbands or fiancés or boyfriends will still love them. For the lone woman, the agonizing question is: will I be able to find someone to love mutilated me?

But Terese Lasser was strong-minded, resourceful. She persistently asked questions, and learned or created answers by herself. A few months later, a woman told her of a mutual acquaintance who had undergone mastectomy and was so deeply depressed she refused to see anyone. She asked Terese Lasser to visit this patient and share some of her own experience.

Mrs. Lasser was reluctant because she hadn't overcome all of her own quandaries. Also, she knew what the woman was going through, and since they weren't close friends, she felt shy about intruding. Nevertheless, she did call the hospital and told the nurse that she had the same kind of operation, by the same surgeon, and wanted to visit the patient to talk to her. Adair, learning of her call, phoned her and approved her visit.

"When I walked into the hospital room a few hours later, I was wearing a formfitting knit dress and my makeup was very carefully applied," Mrs. Lasser wrote. "The nurse left us alone. The woman in bed looked at me . . . when I spoke she did not reply.

"Then I remembered my own feelings, lying in just such a bed."

She began to talk about her experience, and endeavored to reassure the depressed patient about the future. She talked—but received no sign that the woman had heard. Finally, she stood up and said, " 'I'm running late, I've been on the go since seven this morning.' Slowly the patient's head turned on the pillow. I went on. 'A regular merry-go-round! Eighteen holes of golf, then a quick swim, and you can't imagine what it was like driving in here fighting that awful traffic. I'd stay longer but I really must get home to change for a cocktail party.' "

At last the woman began to react. " 'You haven't gone through what I have,' she said. 'They didn't do to you what they've done to me.' "

" 'Yes,' I said. 'Yes, my dear, they did.' "

The woman tried to speak, but no words would come. Finally, she reached for Terese Lasser's hand and pressed it to her cheek. "At that precise moment, I think, the idea for REACH TO RECOVERY was born," Terese Lasser wrote.

The American Cancer Society rehabilitation program known as Reach to Recovery began with reaching out empathically: Mrs. Lasser, a woman recovered from breast-cancer surgery and reestablishing her life, visiting another woman who had just had the operation. Her purpose was to demonstrate by example, and through reassuring words, that life can go on as it was before the operation. This is still the pattern.

Terese Lasser was able to implement her idea because Dr. Adair understood that a visit by a sympathetic woman who had undergone breast surgery might help another patient. It could provide a dimension of care that he, as a man and a busy doctor, could not. Seeing that it worked with one patient, Adair began letting Mrs. Lasser visit others: The moral support she gave through her own presence—always well dressed, well groomed, smiling—made them feel that their cases were not hopeless. They could begin to come to terms with their surgery, see the loss of a breast as a manageable change, not a total disaster.

But more help was needed, physical help as well. With the advice of Dr. Adair, Mrs. Lasser began to develop a set of simple exercises that the patient could begin in the hospital. As time went on, she enlarged and improved on them with the help of doctors, nurses, patients. The act of reaching was the best thing a woman could do to retrain and stretch her muscles—at first just reaching up to brush her hair. Too, self-grooming is the first step to self-respect. Another reaching exercise was simply crumpling paper. Thus began the retraining of muscles cut and sutured during surgery.

Mrs. Lasser also developed a small kit that she could bring to patients as a present. It contained a rubber ball attached to an elastic string. Squeezed in the hand, the ball provided exercise. Later, when the patient had more mobility, the ball could be thrown out and caught as the elastic brought it back. Another exercise, started in the hospital, required reaching out to a wall with the operated arm and walking the fingers up the wall as far as possible without causing severe pain.

The kit also held a plastic-coated rope that could be

thrown over the top of a door to make a kind of pulley; tying tongue depressors as handles to the ends of the rope, and grasping an end in each hand, the patient was instructed to use her unoperated arm to draw the operated arm upward and gradually stretch the muscles.

And there was cosmetic help in the kit: a lightweight breast form for the patient to pin inside her nightgown. Then she could immediately receive visitors looking the way she had before surgery. Mrs. Lasser developed sources for the weightier, permanent prostheses and distributed lists of names and addresses.

Eventually Terese Lasser codified her experience and organized the exercise program into a simple manual with a cheerful yellow cover. Her husband, the late J. K. Lasser, the income tax expert, offered to pay for printing 10,000 copies to be given free to patients. On a visit to Seattle, she showed it to a famous surgeon known to be something of a curmudgeon. He looked at it carefully without expression, then swiveled around in his chair to gaze out the window. Mrs. Lasser sat quietly, expecting the worst. Instead, the great man swiveled back and said, "When can I have three hundred copies?"

With that kind of medical acceptance, Reach to Recovery could begin to reach out all over the country. Mrs. Lasser's personal visits could help only a handful of women; her manual could help hundreds. And it was a passport to the medical profession, as well. She began to talk to doctors' groups, social workers, physiotherapists, and especially nurses. Since almost all nurses were women they could quickly understand the shock and dread of mastectomy patients, and, having close contact they could do the most to help them.

Reach to Recovery began taking over Mrs. Lasser's life. Her correspondence became overwhelming, and her telephone was always busy; her children suggested a private line so they could reach her. Women all over the country wanted to become volunteers, and the movement grew. Reach to Recovery became too much for one person to handle.

Besides, Terese Lasser was not a professional, hence often encountered strong resistance to her visits from doctors and nurses. According to Dr. Holleb, "Many surgeons looked upon the program as interference with the doctor/patient relationship and most felt completely confident that their own patients needed nothing more than their personal physician to meet the total need."

Besides, "Mrs. Lasser was an enthusiastic woman who approached the need for recovery with evangelism. At times she did not seek the approval of the surgeon before visiting a patient in the hospital with her kit and advice," Dr. Holleb said. "As a matter of fact, in the early 1960s when I was an attending surgeon on the breast service of Memorial Sloan-Kettering Cancer Center and associate medical director of the hospital, I personally escorted Mrs. Lasser out the front door of the institution because she was visiting a mastectomy patient without the approval of the responsible surgeon."

Terese Lasser needed professional guidance for her program. It could grow only under the auspices of an accepted, national organization. The logical place to go for help was the American Cancer Society.

In 1969 she contacted Lane Adams, ACS executive vice-president. Adams asked Dr. Holleb to sit in. Holleb was impressed with what Terese Lasser had created, and saw both its value and its potential. He was also aware of how much more had to be done for Reach to Recovery to gain nationwide acceptance among medical professionals.

Dr. Holleb and Dr. William Markel, then vice-president for service and rehabilitation at the ACS, visited Mrs. Lasser's office and started the process of transferring her program to the medical supervision of the ACS. By the end of 1969, it had been merged into the Society. Along with Mrs. Lasser, her volunteers, and her experience, came $90,000 of funds.

Once Reach to Recovery became available through the more than 3,000 units of the ACS, volunteers were selected and trained by doctors and nurses to deal with patients. None was ever visited by a Reach to Recovery volunteer without the surgeon's permission. But even so, Dr. Holleb notes, it was not easy to sell the idea to a great many surgeons. Ultimately this was done, and the program is now so well known that patients often demand to see a volunteer before their surgeons mention it.

The program now includes about 70,000 volunteers in the United States. It has become the largest and best known of the ACS service activities. Its volunteers try to visit every hospitalized breast-cancer patient. In 1983–84, 70,817 women were visited at least once by a Reach to Recovery volunteer, and 41,281 had follow-up visits. Another 15,691 women and their husbands attended Reach to Recovery meetings.

The unmet needs of a single patient were the genesis of a program that has helped hundreds of thousands. It is not easy for physicians and scientists to change the ideas and practices of the medical profession. It is even more difficult for a lay person to penetrate its proud citadel. That Terese Lasser was able to do so proved the truth of her insight and the strength of her determination. Her approach was sometimes more confrontational than sweetly reasonable, but perhaps it takes someone like this to create a working program out of a new and (to professionals) startling idea.

Like other ACS activities, Reach to Recovery attracted interest in foreign countries. Terese Lasser had many overseas correspondents who'd been operated on for breast cancer, and a number wanted to help others like themselves. But volunteers must be carefully selected and trained. This cannot be done by letters or telephone, nor does the program lend itself to a syllabus; it depends on a very intimate personal relationship between visitor and patient. There is no shortage of women who want to volunteer for the work, but not all—in fact only a relative few—have the emotional stability to help others. They must have worked through their own adjustment, psychic as well as physical, before they can try. Hence no volunteer is accepted for Reach to Recovery who has been operated on within the past two years; it takes at least that long to demonstrate physical recovery and personal adjustment.

A few years ago, a young American woman living in Paris had a mastectomy for breast cancer in a private clinic. Mrs. Francine Timothy spoke French fluently, but there was no one to talk to about the trauma of her operation. Like Terese Lasser, she had to invent her own exercises, deal with her own emotional problems, find her own prosthesis.

Returning to the United States, Mrs. Timothy became a Reach to Recovery volunteer. She was as effective in her way as Mrs. Lasser—and her way was quite different: Terese Lasser forged ahead on conviction and zeal; Francine Timothy's natural assets were persuasiveness and charm. She quickly became known in the Society.

The American Cancer Society, in addition to sharing its organizational expertise with other nations, was thinking about making its service programs available internationally as well. Since Reach to Recovery did not exist in an organized fashion outside the United States, it was a possible candidate for export. Because of her American training and her fluent French, it seemed that Francine Timothy might be able to introduce Reach to Recovery into France and perhaps other European countries.

Mrs. Timothy was a foreigner in French society, which outsiders find difficult to penetrate. She was attempting to open a subject that was almost taboo: The French attitude toward cancer in the 1970s was not much different from America's in the early 1900s. And she was a nonprofessional outside the closed world of medicine, which is even more hermetic in France than in the United States.

French surgeons didn't tell their patients that they had cancer. And patients would not acknowledge that they had been treated for it. According to Mrs. Timothy, it was "precancer," and removing a breast was a "preventive" measure. It was impossible to persuade any woman to come forward and admit publicly that she had had a mastectomy. A leg amputation, yes. An arm amputation, yes. A breast amputation—no.

Reach to Recovery has a double meaning in English that is not easily translated. Mrs. Timothy changed the name to Vivre Comme Avant—Live as Before. To get started on patient visits, Mrs. Timothy went to her own surgeon. He gave her permission to visit one of his patients, a Frenchwoman, in the same clinic where she'd had her own surgery. This took great courage on his part, as well as feeling for his patient's needs. The visit proved a success. "And she was so grateful when I left. She told the surgeon," Mrs. Timothy said. He was pleased, and gave her permission to visit other patients. He also spoke to his colleagues.

Mrs. Timothy went to see the director of the Institut Curie, a cancer hospital in Paris, to learn what days and hours would be best (visits are always made outside public visiting hours), how soon after surgery (three or four days: Sooner, the patient is too groggy; later, she has had too much time to sink into depression), and how long the visit should be (fifteen to twenty minutes, thirty minutes at outside, since patients are weak and tired and their attention span is short). Hospitals generally schedule mastectomies on certain days, so it was easy to work out a schedule.

After a year of seeing patients alone in Paris, Mrs. Timothy was invited to a conference of the International Union Against Cancer (UICC) in Monte Carlo, to replace a scheduled speaker who had canceled at the last minute. Following the meeting, Professor Pierre Denoix, head of the prestigious cancer center, the Institut Gustave-Roussy at Villejuif, outside Paris, asked her to join him in a one-hour national television program on breast cancer. The plan was to stage a typical interview with a breast-cancer patient, but despite Dr. Denoit's great reputation, not one patient could be found to admit on TV she'd had a breast removed. Vivre Comme Avant thus had to be described rather than demonstrated. Yet the message came through. As soon as the program ended, the telephone began to ring. Patients all over France wanted help.

From then on, Vivre Comme Avant grew rapidly. Finland heard about it and Mrs. Timothy was invited to that country; and then Ireland. Translated into many languages but having roughly the same meaning, Vivre Comme Avant is is now in fourteen countries outside the United States, and it is different in each, shaped locally by the peoples' attitude toward breast cancer and the prevailing types of treatment.

Wherever Vivre Comme Avant becomes known, it takes root and grows. There are now twenty active volunteers in the Paris area, and in the past twelve years they have seen more than 25,000 patients in that city alone. Throughout France there are forty active chapters.

It is no exaggeration to say that Vivre Comme Avant has helped to reverse the French attitude toward breast cancer. "In the beginning, at least eighty percent of our patients did not know they had the disease," Mrs. Timothy says. "Now, just about one hundred percent know—they tell us proudly, 'My doctor has so much confidence in my emotional stability that he wants me to know what I have; that way I can help him fight it.' "

In recognition of Francine Timothy's contribution to the well-being of French women, in 1981 President Valéry Giscard d'Estaing awarded her the Order of Merit, the highest civilian decoration the French government can confer on a foreigner. Vivre Comme Avant has recently become an official program of the International Union Against Cancer, which will bring it to many countries in Africa and eastern Europe that were outside the ACS sphere.

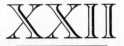

XXII

The Warm Hand of Service to Patients: Volunteers Create Their Own Programs

Through Reach to Recovery and other service activities, the Society extends a warm hand of help and support to nearly a half-million cancer patients a year. This is more than half the cases of newly diagnosed disease.

Every service and rehabilitation program of the ACS has started with the perception of an unfulfilled need among cancer patients or families. It may have begun with an individual or a small group motivated by personal experience or simply by the desire to help others. The initiators may or may not have been American Cancer Society volunteers in the beginning, but eventually their idea developed into a systematic effort that found a natural home within the Society. Its volunteers became, like Terese Lasser, Society volunteers, and their activity attracted others.

INTERNATIONAL ASSOCIATION OF LARYNGECTOMEES (IAL)

There will be about 11,500 new cases of larynx cancer in the United States this year. Of these, 9,500 will occur in men and 2,000 in women. (It's rare in children.)

172

This disease, caused mainly by smoking, is highly curable when detected early. Symptoms are hoarseness and difficulty in swallowing. Treatment of early cases may be minimal, but in about 5,000 U.S. patients each year, it will involve removing the larynx surgically, or irradiating the tumor which may damage vocal cords.

These people require help, usually in the form of speech therapy. They are taught a technique, known as esophageal speech, that requires learning to swallow air and then expel it to cause the esophagus and pharynx to vibrate. The resulting low-pitched sound is shaped by the tongue and mouth to create words, as in normal speech. When laryngectomees (people who have had their larynxes removed) learn to speak this way, they are able to resume their careers and lives.

Since the first operation to remove a human larynx was performed in the 1870s, the problem in dealing with laryngeal cancer became less and less one of survival and more and more one of rehabilitation. As the number of surviving patients grew, several got together and formed a club known as the Lost Chord club in New York City in 1942. Other patients also began forming Lost Chord, and New Voices clubs. Their purpose was mutual assistance, and the main activity was to encourage and teach esophageal speech.

In 1951 Warren H. Gardner, Ph.D., of the Cleveland Hearing and Speech Clinic, had the idea of organizing the clubs into an international organization. This was accomplished at a speech-pathology institute held in Cleveland in 1952. Sponsored jointly by the Cuyahoga Unit of the American Cancer Society, Western Reserve University, and the Vocational Rehabilitation Administration of the Department of Health, Education and Welfare, the International Association of Laryngectomees at first consisted of thirteen clubs.

In 1954 the IAL became a national program of the ACS, with a paid executive secretary and small staff attached to the national ACS office. Today there are 330 member clubs in the United States and eighteen foreign countries: Australia, Belgium, Canada, China, England, Germany, India, Israel, Jamaica, Japan, Korea, Mexico, New Zealand, Scotland, South Africa, Spain, Trinidad, and Venezuela. The *IAL News*, published quarterly, goes to some 38,000 people worldwide, reporting the latest advances in diagnosis, treatment, and speech therapy.

Jack L. Ranney, himself a laryngectomee and former executive director of IAL, said, "One of our jobs is to find people who have lost their larynxes, and don't know about speech therapy. We try to bring them to speech centers. Sometimes we find a man who perhaps hasn't said a word in ten years. You can imagine what it means to him and his family to be able to talk again. And often it means the difference between getting a job, or holding it, and being permanently unemployed."

OSTOMY REHABILITATION PROGRAM

Some patients with intestinal or urinary cancers must have surgery that creates abdominal openings, known as stomas, for the elimination of solid or liquid waste. Such operations create severe emotional and practical problems. The ostomy rehabilitation programs, sponsored by the ACS in cooperation with the United Ostomy Association, offer help to ostomy patients by trained volunteers on a one-to-one basis. Expert enterostomal therapists are also involved in supporting patients through their physical and emotional adjustments.

I CAN COPE

Judi Johnson, a registered nurse in Minneapolis, Minnesota, worked with cancer patients and had friends who had cancer. "In the mid 1970s, I was beginning to see cancer as a chronic illness," she said not long ago. "Patients weren't just dying anymore. Living with cancer was creating a constellation of new problems—adjustment to disease, emotional conflicts that were tearing families apart. My feeling was that much of this stemmed from a sense of loss of control."

Ms. Johnson was not only a nurse but a doctoral student in adult education at the University of Minnesota. She had been working with a group of cancer patients who had sexual problems. To see if it was feasible to broaden this to include other psychosocial difficulties, she studied how these problems were handled in chronic illnesses: diabetes, epilepsy, emphysema, coronary heart disease. She found a common thread: In each case, programs provided what a patient and family needed to know in order to cope with the disease. This obviously could apply to cancer as well.

Johnson volunteered to help cancer patients at the North Memorial Medical Center in Minneapolis. The hospital approved her plan. She worked with a registered nurse on the hospital staff, Pat Norby. They were convinced that the most essential element in cancer treatment was the attitude of the patient, which was generally ignored in health care.

Pat Norby recalls: "I just couldn't believe the anxiety and misinformation the patients had. We, the medical staff, were just not meeting their needs. We couldn't answer all their questions, but we could try to find answers for them."

Adds Judi Johnson: "I CAN COPE [the name of the Johnson-Norby program] is based on the assumption that many worries and anxieties people have can be helped by learning from others in the same boat."

Fifty-four cancer patients were recruited by the hospital and divided into two groups as the first two classes of the I CAN COPE course. The response was enthusiastic. The Minnesota ACS contributed money to develop patient materials, and Gene Sylvestre, a communications specialist, designed the program package materials. He says, "It's a tool for personal change that meets participants where they are and helps them become resourceful. It moves people from asking 'What can I do?' to stating, 'Here's what I can do.' "

In 1977 the president of the Minnesota ACS Division, Dr. Everett Schmidt, made I CAN COPE his presidential project. It was so successful that in 1979 the ACS turned it into a national service and rehabilitation program.

I CAN COPE is cosponsored by the ACS with hospitals and medical centers, and is open without cost to any interested person, with or without cancer. The only requirement is a desire to learn about the disease and how to cope with it. There are no grades, and very little homework. The teachers, known as leaders or facilitators, may be nurses, health educators, social workers.

I CAN COPE has also become international. Ms. Johnson has held workshops in Israel, Australia, the United Kingdom, Sweden, and other countries.

CANSURMOUNT

The idea of CanSurmount is simple and rational: Treated cancer patients help new patients. This parallels Reach to Recovery, the IAL, the Ostomy Clubs. The unique feature of CanSurmount is that the help is not confined to patients having one particular kind of cancer; all kinds are included.

The organization started with a physician and a patient in Denver, Colorado, in 1973. Dr. Paul K. Hamilton, head of oncology at Denver's Presbyterian Medical Center, persuaded Lynn Ringer, a young woman who had recovered from ovarian cancer, to formulate the patient-help program. The plan was to recruit former patients successfully treated for cancer to visit with new patients in the hospital.

CanSurmount was established by the ACS Colorado Division as a new service and rehabilitation program, with Lynn Ringer as state coordinator. Recovered cancer patients were matched with patients currently under treatment, not necessarily by type of cancer but by personality, for compatibility. Their approach was low-key and flexible.

"Listening is the most important part of effective counseling," Dr. Hamilton says. "It requires hearing with all your senses: listening to the patient's words, observing body language, and creating a nonjudgmental atmosphere in which the patient is free to express his or her innermost anxieties and concerns."

To ensure that volunteers are capable of dealing with cancer patients' problems, their own adjustment to the disease is evaluated and such qualities as maturity, responsibility, integrity, and sensitivity are considered. As in all ACS visitation programs, patients are seen only at the request of their physicians. The volunteer visitor later reports informally to the doctor, perhaps identifying problems that a patient may have been reluctant to discuss with the physician.

Relatives, too, are visited and periodically invited to lectures and special events. "We treat the family like another patient," says Dr. Hamilton. "It's a significant part of total care."

The handful of Colorado volunteers who started the program have grown into a force of more than 200. There are now ten CanSurmount chapters in the Denver area and four more throughout the state. The program has spread; there are chapters in 40 ACS divisions.

ROAD TO RECOVERY

Furnishing patients and families with transportation has been part of many ACS service programs. In Massachusetts in 1981, it became a separate statewide activity called "Road to Recovery." The division organized a network of private cars and their volunteer owner-drivers to take cancer patients to treatment facilities. Started in September 1981 with 367 drivers and cars, it more than doubled that number in two years.

In its first year as a Massachusetts Division program,

Road to Recovery carried 1,640 patients to treatments, waited for them, and returned them to their homes, without charge. The average round trip for local treatment was 44.6 miles; treatment at major centers required an average round trip of 148 miles.

Road to Recovery became a national ACS program in 1983, already in force in a number of divisions.

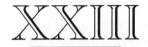

XXIII

Life After Cancer

The management style of Lane Adams celebrated volunteers. He told executives that the ACS role is to encourage volunteer ideas and participation. He deliberately refused the numerous opportunities that naturally come to the head of the ACS to be interviewed by television or the press. These requests arise out of the public's unflagging interest in carcinogens, developments in cancer research, and/or treatment, and their faith in the ACS as a source of objective information. It would have been easier and simpler for him or some staff person to accept the role of Society spokesman, but for twenty-six years, he turned the limelight on volunteers. Giving credit breeds responsibility; and this leads to creativity: volunteers have developed most of the Society's effective service programs.

ACS management has also been creative. Around 1970, Lane Adams was talking with Arthur Holleb about an upcoming medical conference. The Cancer Society has held such conferences for years. They have been credited with increasing physicians' knowledge and awareness of improved methods of diagnosing and treating breast, lung, colon/rectum, and other forms of cancer. Because of medical progress, the number of cancer cures had been rising steadily for decades, and the life span of patients who could not be cured had been greatly lengthened. The number of Americans who had been diagnosed for cancer five years earlier and were still alive had risen to between 3 and 4 million.

179

"Why not have a conference that focuses on the cancer patient in areas other than medicine?" Adams asked Holleb. "It could deal with the psychological problems, the social problems, the employment problems, the emotional problems—facing death, helping with the family. We could call it the 'Human Values Conference.' "

Holleb was receptive. He knew from his associate, Dr. William Markel, then vice-president for service and rehabilitation, that the need for service was increasing exponentially. The time had come to focus public and professional attention on this trend, which mirrored a truly profound change in the cancer picture. There had never been a national meeting of the type Adams proposed. Just holding it would be a way of making a statement.

Consistent with Adams's policies, the organizing committee was made up of volunteers, including several ACS directors and the 1971–72 president, Dr. A. Hamblin Letton, of Atlanta, Georgia. The only staff person on the committee was Dr. Holleb; the staff coordinator was Dr. Markel. Dr. Benjamin F. Byrd, Jr., an ACS delegate director later to become president of the Society, was chairman.

The Human Values Conference was held in Atlanta, on June 22–24, 1972. Seven hundred people attended, representing all of the disciplines, professions, and businesses dealing with the many problems of cancer patients and their families other than diagnosis and treatment.

Lane Adams gave the opening address:

> There's a new excitement in the ranks of the American Cancer Society today because we know the direction our efforts must take to make life better for the cancer patient. Lives are being saved from cancer—but we must ask ourselves if they are worth living.
>
> Human values really mean the sense of worth and security that comes from having a job; the joy of being loved and esteemed; the essential ingredient called hope.
>
> Too often the cancer patient is alone with crushing fears.

His family is afraid to mention the word *cancer*. The American Cancer Society . . . can teach people the value of expressing their feelings. . . . We must emphasize that dignity is always possible. We can help the child with cancer, we can help families under emotional stress.

. . . Our volunteers must remind business that cancer patients can be fine workers and active professionals before the five-year survival mark.

Asked Dr. Byrd:

Are patients any the worse physically for their bout and victory with cancer? Aren't they thoroughly employable people? One thinks so. And hopes so. And then one hears . . . "I'm sorry. I'm afraid you wouldn't fit in."

Theoretically at least, the person who has a good chance of winning over cancer should be happy indeed. He or she has an opportunity to live. But all too often survival is itself a problem.

What kind of survival? That's what the patient worries about. Will I be able to go back to normal living? Do the things I did before? Or am I going to have to hide at home?

The conference heard from forty-nine speakers. A former patient and professional writer, Herbert Black, described what it meant to have cancer, as did the well-known singer Marguerite Piazza. Physicians, a clergyman, an educator spoke about what to tell the patient, how to deal with nonverbal communication, and how to handle the ever-present problem of quackery. Other topics were "Adaptation to Cancer: The Return to Society," "The Child with Cancer," "The Patient and the American Cancer Society." The latter included information on homemaking counseling, gift and loan closets, and other services available through ACS.

In summing up, Dr. Holleb said:

A Conference such as this places in proper perspective the importance of compassion, the need for sympathy and the true worth of consideration for other human beings.

The existentialist believes that life is meaningless—that it is not to be cherished—unless one acts. Most of us here would agree with this philosophy. I am sure that the papers presented at this conference provoked thought—hopefully they will provoke action as well.

The conference launched a new concept: that there is indeed life after cancer. This presented a host of new problems that were being dealt with only sporadically and fragmentarily. The meeting informed the public and got the professionals thinking and moving in new directions.

Lane Adams continued to push this new Society initiative. He found strong support in the 1976–77 ACS president, Dr. Benjamin F. Byrd, Jr. Together, they oversaw the organization of a second ACS conference on human values and cancer. Held in Chicago on September 7–9, 1977, and vibrating with the energy unleashed by the first, it attracted more than twice as many professionals, business people, and lay volunteers, 1,700 in all.

Dr. Holleb again summed up:

All of us want to live with dignity and respect, not merely to exist. We must, therefore, devote as much energy to preserving psychic integrity in patients as to physiological integrity. This conference taught us that an "ego prosthesis" must be offered to cancer patients. Given hope, people can cope; the clergy can act as a psychic broker to the physician and a link to the community.

A third conference on the same subject was held in Washington, D.C., in April 1980, attended by more than 1,900 people. The Fourth Human Values Conference took place in March 1984 in New York City.

There can be little doubt that the lives of many if not most U.S. cancer patients have been greatly ameliorated as a result of the information and attitudes spread through these meetings, and the new research and training they engendered.

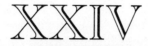

XXIV

Affirmative Action: Cancer in Minorities

During Lane Adams's tenure as executive vice-president of the ACS, there were a number of basic policy changes and initiatives. Perhaps none of them is more important than the major shift in the Society's perspective regarding minorities.

The ASCC had been established by white males, although several were actually recruited by a white female (Mrs. Mead). And although the ACS changed directions and policies many times over the years, the national organization, probably without deliberate intent, remained a kind of Caucasian club. The ACS was not unique in this respect at that time.

As usual, change began out where the Society was in direct contact with communities. Perhaps the key event took place in Washington, D.C. three years after Lane Adams took charge. It involved a young black surgeon, Dr. LaSalle D. Leffall, Jr., who had graduated from and been trained in surgery at Howard University in D.C. in the early 1950s, and later became a senior oncological surgical fellow at Memorial Sloan-Kettering Hospital in New York. In 1962 he returned to Howard as professor of surgery, and volunteered for the District of Columbia Division of the American Cancer Society.

Although the city of Washington was 75 percent black, there were only three other blacks—all physicians—in the D.C. Division: Drs. Paul Cornelia, Robert Jason, and Jack White.

> Dr. Leffall recalled recently: We devised a committee on community involvement, a euphemism for minorities. I was chairman; the idea was to let people know that the ACS wasn't just research, or just white middle-class conservatives. That was how many of my colleagues had characterized it, and they asked why I joined. I told them, "Well, if it's like that, maybe we ought to try to do something to change it."

Dr. Leffall and his associates began studying the special problems of the D.C. area, which meant largely those of blacks and cancer. He found his white associates in the division receptive. "It was the right time, the 1960s," Dr. Leffall said recently. "Somebody told me that if I'd come in ten years earlier, no way would we have changed their thinking. But there had been the march on Washington, and attitudes were in a ferment."

Dr. Leffall not only came along at the right time, he was the right man. Handsome, eloquent, relaxed, he is very easy to like and began to be noticed early on. He was invited to speak at the Hawaii Division, the first of scores of speeches he was to give. His favorite subject: medical progress against cancer.

By 1970 Leffall had been elected a member of the national board of directors, where he displayed unmistakable leadership qualities. Dr. Holleb, who had known Leffall at Memorial Hospital, arranged for him to join the Audiovisual Committee, whose job was to analyze educational films. When it was quickly seen that he had an incisive mind and made creative suggestions, he was given other, increasingly responsible committee assignments. This is the process by which the ACS indoctrinates and advances volunteer leaders. Dr. Leffall did not know it, but he was being groomed for one of the two highest professional volunteer offices in the ACS, the presidency.

He also continued to impress his fellow volunteers in the District of Columbia. In 1970 they elected him president of the D.C. Division—the first black officer of that division. That year the National Cancer Institute issued a report affirming what Dr. Leffall and his colleagues had been finding in their community: increased morbidity and mortality from cancer among black Americans, as compared with Caucasians.

Meanwhile, in 1969 a parallel change began to take place on the ACS staff. John Henry Jones, then fifty-one, joined the Society's national office as news editor. There should have been nothing remarkable about this—Mr. Jones had been a news editor of the weekly *Medical World News*—except that he was the first black executive hired by the national office.

Like Dr. Leffall, a very friendly and outgoing person, Jones immediately proved that the Society's slogan—"You can make a difference"—was true. His very presence brought a new outlook. Suddenly many realized that the ACS national organization had had only limited contact with a large segment of the American people, the minorities.

Jones was an effective editor and publicist. He set up the first ACS list of black press representatives. He began talking about the Society's broadening its perspective. He knew from personal observation that the cancer problems in the black community were different from those among whites. But all ACS materials were addressed to whites. He suggested that two films be made specifically for black women, on breast cancer and uterine cancer. These were produced by the ACS Public Education Department around 1971: *Time Out for Life* and *Five Minutes of Breast Self-Examination*.

Jones also requested that Lawrence Garfinkel and Edwin Silverberg, of the Society's Epidemiological and Statistical Department, supply statistics on cancer among black Americans to supplement the standard annual Society publication, *Cancer Facts & Figures*. He issued a fact sheet of such information annually, helping to make the public-information media aware that there were serious differences between black and white Americans in cancer incidence and survival.

At the 1972 ACS Science Writers' Seminar, March 24–29 at Clearwater Beach, Florida, a typical Jones press release emphasized that death rates from cancer of the esophagus had been reported rising steadily among black Americans. Several studies had shown that there might be a link between higher incidence of this disease and heavy drinking of alcoholic beverages, and with syphilis. Dr. T. W. Roberts, chief of pathology at Harlem Hospital in New York City, noted as the result of a ten-year study that "there is some connection between the low economic status of these patients and their condition," and that "in certain dietary or cultural patterns . . . the inference is definite."

Over several years John Jones helped broaden the contact between the American Cancer Society and blacks and other minorities. Meanwhile, Dr. Leffall was moving up the ladder of important committee assignments, which included Service and Rehabilitation, Professional Education, Medical and Scientific. These would culminate in the vice-presidency and presidency—a five-year process in all.

In 1977 Jones and Mrs. Agnes J. Dixon, a black woman who had earned a number of promotions in the ACS national office and was then executive asssistant to Dr. Holleb, spoke to Lane Adams about the minority community. He asked them to put their suggestions in writing. They did, as follows:

> All of us are aware of the difficulties in reaching minority populations with ACS messages as well as motivating their involvement in the total ACS program. The ACS record in pioneering the involvement of minority peoples in the cancer control fight is substantial. Compared to other health agencies, we lead in this area, although the immensity of the problem calls for more action.
>
> A study of various programs for the past ten years will show the successes and difficulties in reaching the targeted populations.

As examples, they listed a dozen programs in as many Divisions between 1962 and 1976. These included a cervical cancer program among blacks in Maryland; a Mexican-American health project in Fresno, California; and annual checkups for Sioux Indians in South Dakota.

"Thus, the basic apparatus for reaching minority peoples in the control of cancer and the mechanism for enlistment of their support into Crusade already exists," they wrote.

The populations they wanted to reach included 24,700,000 blacks (they pointed out that the black American community is highly organized, with leaders, exemplars, and trend setters, and institutions), 6,600,000 Mexican Americans, nearly 2 million Puerto Ricans, close to 800,000 American Indians, and 700,000 Cuban Americans.

Adams asked them to speak to Dr. Leffall, who had been giving him similar information. Out of this visit came the suggestion for a national conference to be held in New York City in February 1979, entitled "Meeting the Challenge of Cancer Among Black Americans."

Meanwhile, the "making of the president" process for Dr. Leffall had culminated: He was installed at the 1978 annual national meeting in November of that year. Dr. Leffall was also asked to chair the first black national cancer conference.

It took place on February 15–17, 1979, in Washington, D.C. Four hundred people attended, among them representatives of fifty-five black American civic, religious, fraternal, labor, and scientific organizations, from thirty-two ACS divisions. It was the beginning of a creative partnership between the ACS and minorities.

The conference opened with Miss Lena Horne, the well-known singer, introducing Vernon E. Jordan, Jr., then president of the National Urban League. Mr. Jordan pointed out that the incidence of some cancers is twice as high in blacks as in whites, and that survival rates were lower among blacks.

Lane Adams announced a special allocation of $250,000 to recruit and train black American professionals for the ACS, to "help people help each other control cancer," and $100,000 for follow-up activities to the black conference.

Among the black leaders who spoke were Dr. Sidney J. Cutler, professor of community and family health at the Georgetown School of Medicine; Dr. Harold P. Freeman, director of surgery at New York's Harlem Hospital; Janice Kissner, president of the Zeta Phi Beta sorority; Dr. Louis W. Sullivan, dean and director of the School of Medicine, Morehouse College, Atlanta, Georgia; Jonathan Comer of the United Steel Workers; and Carrie Rogers, president of the National Black Nurses Association.

Dr. Leffall, in his closing address, said, "We must meet the challenge of cancer among black Americans. Our local units and divisions know this is a major goal of the Society. We believe our course is just, our charge is real, our commitment is true, our course is set. There can be no turning back."

On May 17–18, 1979, a follow-up workshop that asked that a national advisory committee on cancer in black Americans be appointed to report directly to the ACS National Board of Directors; and that members should include the Hispanic community. The ACS National Committee on Minorities and Cancer was chaired by Dr. Harold Freeman.

A communications advisory committee came up with the idea for the first national survey of black attitudes toward, and knowledge of, cancer.

The study was done by EVAXX, Inc., a black organization, directed by Dr. John J. Cardwell. It employed standard sampling techniques and was concentrated in the urban population, since some 85 percent of U.S. blacks live in cities.

The survey found the following:

- Although black Americans were more likely than whites to get cancer, 73 percent of blacks consistently underestimated their cancer incidence. They believed that cancer was a "white man's disease," when in fact cancer incidence among black American males had climbed 36 percent between 1947 and 1969, but only 6.7 percent among white U.S. males.

• Blacks were twice as fatalistic as whites about cancer: Only 20 percent believed that as many as one-third of cancer patients survived for five years.

• Only 69 percent of blacks knew that a lump in the breast might mean cancer; they were aware of lung cancer, but knew little of colorectal, prostate, and esophageal tumors.

• Blacks were apathetic about most cancer symptoms, except bleeding. But 84 percent wanted to know more about the disease.

However, as Dr. Freeman noted,

The black population is comprised of a high number of poor people with a relatively low educational level. Their priorities are food, shelter and the avoidance of crime. In the absence of pain or bleeding—usually signs of late cancer—many fail to seek medical help.

. . . A poor person typically experiences great difficulty in entering the health-care system. Not able to pay for a private physician, the poor patient is frequently seen first in an emergency room and referred to a clinic. Long waiting lines and complex registration procedures are common. A minimally symptomatic patient is likely to be discouraged when faced by a lengthy process of diagnosis. . . . The result is often late diagnosis in an incurable state. . . .

Dr. Freeman called for affirmative action in health care. "The most dramatic improvement in cancer mortality achievable in the light of current knowledge would occur if the survival of poor people with cancer were raised to that of the middle class and affluent," he wrote.

A second conference, this time embracing all U.S. minorities, was held by the ACS in April 1983 in Memphis,

Tennessee. Special focus was on the six major ethnic groups in the United States: Alaskan natives, American Indians, Asians, black Americans, Hispanics, and Polynesians. Great progress has been made within the American Cancer Society as the result of the minority conferences and the presidency of Dr. Leffall:

- The number of black, Hispanic, and Asian professionals on the ACS staff more than trebled in four years, from about 50 in 1979 to 180 in 1983.

- There were ten national board members from minority groups in 1983, as against less than half that number in 1979. The 58 divisions had 353 minority members of boards of directors, including three board chairmen, one president, one Executive Committee chairman, and four committee chairmen.

- Important advances have been made in extending ACS programs into black, Hispanic, and other communities.

Dr. Leffall devoted nearly all of his time to the Society during the year of his presidency—probably more than any other president. He traveled twelve to twenty days every month; in his busiest month he was on the move for twenty-nine days. He visited fifty of the fifty-eight divisions, some more than once, and covered a total of more than 300,000 miles between November 1978 and November 1979. ACS invitations took precedence over everything else, except seeing patients and performing surgery.

"You've got to remember that every man's time on Earth is finite," he said. "What you hope is to do something that will make it easier for those who follow. I know I couldn't have accomplished anything without those who came before, and I hope that I have made the path a little easier for those who come after."

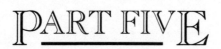

PART FIVE

Public and Private Issues

XXV

Crusade

If volunteer power is the engine of the American Cancer Society, it is self starting and makes its own fuel: ACS volunteers finance their activities through their annual Cancer Crusade, which is simultaneously a public-education effort and a fund-raiser.

The Crusade is probably the largest volunteer health-related activity in the world. The drive involves more ACS volunteers than any other of the Society's programs: about 1,600,000 each year. Almost all of them visit neighbors, door-to-door.

Its title fittingly sums up the attitude of the Society: The fight against cancer is imbued with an almost religious fervor for the majority of ACS volunteers. The quasi-military concept implicit in the name is traceable, as well, to the Women's Field Army.

Started in 1945 by professional fund-raisers who were paid by the Laskers, the Crusade has been staffed ever since by volunteers, guided by in-house fund-raising experts. It has consistently outdone itself year after year since 1945, when it began with more than $4 million ($4,292,491.56), through 1985, when it topped $243 million. There was only one year, 1960 when income declined, though by less than a million dollars, the year when the ACS severed its connections with the United Way–Community Chest drives. Overall, from 1945 to 1985 inclusive, the Crusade has raised $2,946,000,000 for ACS cancer-control programs and administration.

It is unique among fund-raising drives because its campaign handbill, known as the mass-distribution leaflet, does not mention or request money. It is always an educational piece, accenting some aspect of cancer prevention or safeguard. Some 35 million were printed this year on about five railroad-carloads of paper, making it one of the largest editions of any nongovernment document in the United States.

The drive starts in January with an event known as the national Kickoff, which brings together outstanding volunteers from all over the country for a one-day meeting to spark the volunteers. It's a kind of pep rally, with star actors and entertainers, such as Gregory Peck and Lawrence Welk, who volunteer as crusade leaders, and with updates from doctors and scientists. There are usually one or two personal appeals from recovered cancer patients. In 1985, for example, Jeff Blatnick, the champion U.S. amateur wrestler, told how he had overcome Hodgkin's disease and gone on to win an Olympic gold medal in 1984. Blatnick later had a recurrence of cancer which was again put into remission.

The Crusade is a year-round activity, but its peak is the month of April, designated by Congress as "Cancer Control Month." Every U.S. president, starting with Franklin D. Roosevelt, has issued a special proclamation announcing the Crusade theme. In 1986 it was "Hand in Hand," as contrasted with the theme of the first Crusade in 1945, which pictured three children over the caption "They All Had Cancer." The implication was that all three had died, which indeed was what happened.

Each U.S. president, starting with Richard M. Nixon, has invited the American Cancer Society leadership to the White House before the Crusade and presented the Courage Award of the Society to a cured cancer patient. In 1985 President Ronald Reagan presented the award to Jeff Keith, a twenty-two-year-old athlete who lost a leg to osteogenic sarcoma, a bone cancer, ten years ago. Mr. Keith, who said he was "challenged, not handicapped" by his artificial leg, ran

3,200 miles across the United States to demonstrate that cancer can be beaten. He ran through seventeen states and the District of Columbia, starting in Boston on June 4, 1984, and ending in Los Angeles on February 18, 1985. Previous Courage Award winners were Amanda Blake, actress; Gene Littler, golfer; and Otto Graham, football player.

The Crusade, whose main activity is door-to-door solicitation, is considered the portal through which most volunteers enter the Cancer Society. Many go on to undertake more important responsibilities; two recent chairmen of the board of directors, G. Robert Gadberry (Wichita, Kansas)—who took over the executive vice-presidency after Lane Adams— and Allan K. Jonas (Los Angeles, California), both started as Crusade volunteers, as did the current national secretary, Mrs. Lawrence J. (Kathleen) Horsch of Minneapolis, Minnesota.

The celebrities who participate in the Crusade often give a great deal of their time and energy. Gregory Peck, for example, interrupted a busy career to visit twenty-six of the Society's division meetings in that many states. Each such visit usually takes one or two days. Lawrence Welk, who was Crusade chairman in 1968 and again in 1973, used his network television program to launch appeals for the Crusade and started the donations off with a large one of his own. Recruited originally by Matty Rosenhaus, president of J. B. Williams Company, who owned his show, Welk became deeply involved with the Society and would visit division kickoffs. A staff member recalls him dancing with every woman volunteer who wished to dance at the Maryland Division kickoff in the 1960s.

Two celebrity volunteers have notable records of perennial service to the ACS Crusade. One is Virginia Graham, the TV talk show hostess, who went public with the news of her cure of endometrial cancer in the 1950s, a time when few people would acknowledge that they had had cancer. Miss Graham is still touring the country making speeches about cancer after more than twenty years of ACS volunteer work.

The other was the late Bill Gargan, who consecrated the last twenty years of his life for the ACS. A star of movies, theater, and television, in 1960 Gargan was playing the role of an ex-president dying of cancer in a West Coast production of Gore Vidal's *The Best Man* when he contracted a persistent sore throat. He had a checkup, and later recalled the doctor's no-nonsense approach: "You've got cancer of the larynx,' he said. Just like that. It jolted me right down to my socks. 'What's the procedure?' I asked. 'We operate, you live,' he said. 'We don't operate, you die.' "

Gargan had his operation, and then learned esophageal speech so well that he was able to give thousands of fund-raising talks for the ACS until his death at age of seventy-four in 1979. Gargan, who traveled an average of 250,000 miles a year for the ACS, is credited with raising many millions of dollars for cancer control.

Two well-known TV personalities of the 1950s and 1960s, Ed Sullivan ("The Ed Sullivan Show") and Ralph Edwards ("This Is Your Life"), were Crusade chairmen who had a large impact. Since their shows were owned by corporations, they were free to plug the Crusade; now shows are network-owned or controlled, and plugs are forbidden.

Other recent Crusade chairmen who gave generously of their time are Cliff Robertson, John Forsythe, Kirk Douglas, Danny Kaye, Amanda Blake, Ann Landers, Raquel Welch, Peter Graves, and the late Marvella Bayh.

It is impossible to participate in any Crusade and not be impressed with the zeal of the volunteers. It is also impossible, and certainly unfair to the millions who have participated in Crusades during the past forty years, to pick one or a group of volunteers as the best. But few would deny that one who was truly outstanding (and still active in his eighties) is Arch Avery, an Atlanta banker.

Mr. Avery took on the Crusade chairmanship of the Georgia Division in 1963–64. Participation made him alert to the seven warning signals, and sent him to the doctor with bowel symptoms. He was unsatisfied with a negative finding, and continued to seek further tests and opinions until he was diagnosed and operated on successfully for colorectal cancer. Thus, he credited his Crusade involvement with saving his life.

An enthusiastic public speaker and creative promoter, Avery became a gung-ho activist about cancer checkups. He toured southeastern states, asking manufacturers to give presents to people who could certify that they had had complete cancer checkups, including the examination that patients disliked and doctors often avoided: the proctosigmoidoscopy—examination of the lower bowel by an uncomfortable rigid tube some twenty-five centimeters long (about ten inches). Hundreds of southerners got suits of clothes and radios, donated by manufacturers, for undergoing checkups, and not a few unsuspected cancers were found and treated.

In recent years Crusade income has been supplemented by a growing number of special events, which can be golf tournaments (there is a national series that used to be known as the Walter Hagen Tournaments), fashion shows, hog-calling contests, costume balls, or anything local sponsors can dream up. A few years ago such events were not always favorably regarded, especially in New York, where some high-society sponsors rented a ship and took it outside the twelve-mile limit for legal gambling. The proceeds went to the Crusade, but the gambling offended some people. *Time* magazine published a critical article, to which Dr. Eugene Pendergrass, Society president, responded, "We'll take the devil's money to do the Lord's work."

Crusade remains the core activity of the ACS. "A division that does well in Crusade is almost invariably one where all programs are well run and successful," Lane Adams noted. "It's the best test for volunteer motivation and participation I know."

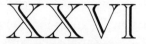

XXVI

United Way or a
Better Way?

When Lane Adams joined the Society's staff in 1959, two potentially divisive policy disagreements were being fought out in units and divisions from coast to coast, as well as in the national board of directors. Each threatened schism and defection from the Society, and one did in fact tear large holes in its fabric.

The first of these controversies involved the United Way of America, an organization created out of "community chests," local unified fund-raising drives in hundreds of towns and cities throughout the United States. They were organized to support a number of local charities. Approximately 350 ACS units had joined in community-chest fund-raising, accounting for some 15 percent of Society income. When the community chests joined under the national umbrella of United Way, this affected the independence of those ACS units involved.

The great majority of ACS units did not belong to United Way, which was expanding into many more towns and cities. In some ACS regions the boards of directors voted against permitting units to affiliate with any new community chests, while those already affiliated were allowed to continue.

"This created much dissension," recalls Francis J. Wilcox, former chairman of the ACS National Board. "One unit would be working all alone to raise money, and they'd look over at another town where the ACS belonged to the

Community Chest and didn't have to work so hard. They didn't like that."

This was happening to many parts of the country, and pressure from the grass roots forced the national board of directors to consider the problem. After checking five years of records, they found that in comparable communities, "those in United Way were raising only half as much money as those that remained independent," says Thomas Ulmer of Jacksonville, Florida, who has served at all levels of the ACS including as board chairman. "More important, we were not getting our education message across, being merged with forty or fifty other local organizations. The central purpose of our Crusade is not just to raise money but to help save lives. The United Way is designed to make it easy to give one time a year to all philanthropies."

"Our studies proved that where units belonged to community chests, there was little growth," Mr. Wilcox adds. "Unaffiliated units were growing much faster. Besides, when you were one organization among many in a pool, fighting before a budget committee for your allocation, you were competing with hungry children, or widows who needed support. That was no position for the Cancer Society to be in."

The question came down to whether the ACS should continue to belong to United Way or go it alone. The debate was long and acrimonious. At last, in 1959, the ACS National Board voted to drop out of the United Way. This meant giving up more than $4 million of assured income that year.

The ACS is the fortunate focus of enormous volunteer dedication, not only in numbers but in commitment. People volunteer to work for the Society because they want to wipe out cancer. Their Crusade efforts are pointed toward that.

When people with that kind of commitment are merged into an organization whose interest is overall community service and whose expertise is mainly fund-raising, their motivation is blurred if not lost, and their involvement diminishes.

However, the ACS was (and is) no monolith. Within any voluntary organization large enough to span this continent, there must be many diverse, sometimes opposing, regional and local interests. For example, many small towns were much less dependent on United Way than were large cities. Detroit, in particular, was a big United Way entity. The automobile companies opened their work force to a single United Way solicitation a year; they couldn't afford the time for many separate drives. Walter Reuther, president of the United Automobile Workers of America, supported management's position on United Way, as did the AFL-CIO unions.

The Society's Wayne County (Detroit) unit had received especially favored treatment—$750,000 a year from United Way. The motor community was astounded that the ACS would turn its back on that kind of support when it needed funds for cancer research. The Detroit press judged that dropping out of the Torch Fund, the local United Way, was a selfish act, prompted by sinister motives. As a result, the ACS was the target of bad publicity in Detroit.

There and throughout the neighboring states of Indiana, Pennsylvania, and Ohio, ACS units that belonged to United Way threatened to secede from the Society. Recalls Frank Wilcox:

> The United Way wanted to retain them as part of its drive, and offered to fund them as independent cancer organizations if they seceded. I went out there with Dr. Lowell Coggeshall to try to persuade them to stay with ACS. But some did drop out; they still exist as "Red Doors" [fund-raising units]. They have, of course, since been replaced by ACS units.
>
> But the major dropout was Detroit. They left the ACS, even though the unit president stayed with the Society. There is still a cancer foundation in Detroit unaffiliated with the ACS, financed by the Torch Fund, that runs its own cancer research and control program. It took some years before the ACS could replace its Detroit units.
>
> And where we did keep our units, we often lost about half the board of directors, the business half. Those people were

with corporations that took part in United Way. So we had to rebuild our local boards, a long, slow process. It was a very traumatic time for the Society.

And it was costly as well. ACS Crusade income, which had risen steadily since the reorganization in 1945, dropped during Lane Adams's first year on the job.

ACS CRUSADE INCOME

1957–58: $29,796,000
1958–59: $30,372,000
1959–60: $28,356,000
1960–61: $30,791,000
1961–62: $33,313,000

During the period 1959–60, the Society had a net drop in income of about $2 million. And there was the additional lost revenue that probably would have accrued had the organization continued its steady annual increases.

But as the figures show, even on a strictly financial basis the judgment that took ACS out of United Way proved correct. Within the year when severance took place, the ACS reduction in income was less than the amount of United Way contributions. The loss was only about 6 percent of previous income, or less than half the $4 million dollars expected from United Way. In other words, ACS volunteers were able to replace half the United Way income during the first year the Society dropped out of that organization. This appeared to be the result of renewed zeal on the part of people working solely for the organization they treasured. And ACS income began rising much faster a year after the split.

However, donations, are only one measure of the organization's vitality. Said Lane Adams recently:

When you were receiving money with little effort, there is a tendency to sit on your hands, and account only for the spending, not the generating of funds.

I think that withdrawing from United Way resulted in a determination by our volunteers to work harder. It forced the Society to expand its volunteer corps, train them better—they did the job. It strengthened the Society.

The traumas of defections to United Way began to heal in a few years. But there was a fair residue of dislike for the Society in many areas where units had seceded, or where the community-chest spirit was strong. Standing aside from this communal philanthropy, the ACS was often perceived by corporate America as self-serving, arrogant. And this attitude was reflected in local media, loyal to the "give once for all" community charity.

On its side, United Way sorely missed the Society. The ACS national reputation and the appeal of its programs had been an important support, helping to carry a host of less well-known local causes.

For these reasons, United Way made repeated efforts over the next fifteen years to bring the Society back into affiliation.

Adams felt obliged to listen to their offers. Cooperating with United Way could help improve the ACS's image in many areas. More important, it would clear the way to ACS in-plant educational programs. The Society offers direct, immediate lifesaving and health-improvement information through its films, filmstrips, and lectures by physicians and nurses on such vital subjects as breast cancer and quitting smoking. These programs appeal to large audiences, but without United Way, they could not reach employees in the vast majority of large businesses and industries.

United Way is usually the only philanthropy permitted to solicit funds in these places. Too, employees can contribute to the United Way via payroll deductions. This checkoff makes giving both "official" and painless, and almost guarantees income. In Lane Adams's judgment, however, "there was no way we could submit to a review of our needs by local United Way allocations committees: it didn't fit our national program requirements."

The ACS wasn't primarily interested in the extra revenue; its Crusade income had been growing fast every year since it left United Way. In 1974 it received more than $73 million—about two and one-half times the amount raised in 1961. Other sources of revenue—legacies, bequests, memorials—were adding greatly to the total. In 1961 the ACS had received over $6 million in bequests; in 1974 this had risen to more than $24 million.

At about that time, a new executive director joined United Way: William Aramony. He insisted on meeting with Lane Adams. After several meetings Adams was convinced that "he knew if we were ever to have any kind of agreement, it would have to take into account some of our inalienable rights."

There were several reasons why both sides wanted to get together. "People in industry needed our educational programs, and we needed their involvement and support," said Adams. Furthermore, United Way was under attack from various activist groups as giving too little help to minority causes. Affiliation with the well-liked American Cancer Society could help deflect such criticism.

Early in 1974, William Aramony and an assistant, Robert Beggan; met with Lane Adams and Richard P. McGrail, deputy executive vice-president of the ACS. On a blackboard, Aramony drew two columns of issues and principles: In one were those possible of accommodation; in the other, things that could not be changed. These were finally organized into a document that could become a *pro forma* contract between an ACS unit and a local United Way chapter.

Essentially, the contract would permit the ACS to continue its own door-to-door Cancer Crusade while giving it entry into plants and offices for educational campaigns; and would give the Society a guaranteed percentage of United Way's payroll deductions.

This arrangement would create special status for the ACS. Untied Way would have to change its bylaws to accommodate it, but the ACS did not have to change its bylaws.

"Aramony's neck was way out on this," Adams recalled, "as was mine. We were negotiating without authority, in contravention of established policies of our two organizations. He was criticized by his various executives around the country, as I was, and still am by some. We were both, you might say, out of sync with parts of our constituencies."

Allan Jonas, later to become board chairman of the ACS, was chairman of the Crusade Committee. Adams asked if he could bring a visitor to a committee meeting in November 1974. "I told Mr. Jonas who it was—Aramony; he was skeptical but thought it might be interesting."

Adams had confidence in Aramony's ability to present a clear case, and in fact the latter was very articulate and candid before the committee. Nevertheless,

> . . . after the meeting, people came up to me and said "Have you lost your head?" Adams recalled. A number didn't appreciate that I'd invited the enemy into the family circle. There was great concern whether Aramony was really sincere and honest. But some executives in our largest divisions were willing to listen. One of the early ones was Curt Reiman, executive vice-president of the Texas Division, who had made a limited agreement with United Way in 1976 [permitted under ACS rules if restricted to business and industry]. In 1978 United Way changed its constitution and bylaws to meet national ACS requirements.

United Way surveys showed that its donors would give more, and more donors would give, if they were supporting health organizations. And United Way knew from experience in sharing government employees' payroll deductions with the American Cancer Society, where donors were able to choose the recipients of their deductions, that the Society received more than 50 percent of such donations. In their words, the ACS brought "card value" to the partnership.

In 1979, a year's experience proved that the ACS had been able to mount scores of large, successful educational events in business and industry. As an example, in a demonstration breast self-examination project at the General Mills Company in Minneapolis, Minnesota, 86 percent of the company's female employees participated. This was a large new audience for ACS public education.

All contracts were made directly between ACS divisions or units and United Way chapters. All were carefully limited in scope and time, under specific guidelines. All were easily cancelable. Where the new contracts were made, regular Society fund-raising activities—residential Crusade; special events; special gifts, legacies, and memorials—continued to prosper, and units and divisions received additional moneys through United Way from previously untapped business and industry sources.

In 1980 the ACS board formally spelled out the authority to make new agreements with United Way limited to solicitation in business, industry and/or government. Currently there are about 110 such limited contracts in force, and they bring in about $20 million a year to the ACS, less than 10 percent of current income. In general, these new partnerships have been satisfactory to both organizations, and their number has continued to grow, although there remain opponents to the arrangement on both sides.

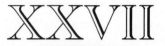

XXVII

". . . Without Representation"

The arguments over United Way brought to the surface another ACS organizational problem that had been festering during the 1950s. There was a national board of about sixty directors-at-large, theoretically representing all parts of the ACS; there were also regional directors, one from each of seven regions into which the country was divided. Regional assemblies, representing these regions' divisions, each selected a single director to the national board.

"It was like the early days in the United States," recalls Frank Wilcox, "when the state legislatures elected U.S. senators. The divisions felt that they were shortchanged in this arrangement."

This resulted partly from a number of organizational anomalies, a heritage of uneven development of the ACS. Some regions represented as few as three statewide divisions, while others had as many as nine. "This led to some of the divisions not having any direct representation on the Board of Directors for a number of years," wrote Dr. Thomas Carlile, in 1983. Dr. Carlile was 1961–62 president of the ACS and is currently director of the breast-cancer research project at the Virginia Mason Research Center in Seattle, Washington. "As a result, there was increasing agitation for some more equitable system."

"As the Society grew," recalls Wilcox, "there was a perception that the important decisions gravitated toward the national board. A kind of grass-roots movement sprang up in the Southwest and Midwest divisions, based on the feeling that they were being screened off. They wanted direct representation of divisions on the National Board."

Wrote Dr. Carlile:

In 1959, President Warren Cole first appointed a committee to study the reorganization of the Society to answer this need. Dr. Eugene Pendergrass was the chairman of this committee, which held many meetings and hearings. Some members of the Society argued that the existing form of organization had progressed very rapidly in programming and fund-raising to become one of the most prestigious voluntary health agencies in the country. Others felt that progress would be even more rapid with so-called direct divisional representation (DDR). Several plans were presented over the two years of study, including proportional representation, based upon either:

1. fund-raising capability, with additional delegates or directors for Divisions raising over $1 million and more for those raising in excess of $2.5 million, or,

2. additional proportional representation depending upon population.

The Pendergrass Committee polled each Division on its views. A progress report was given at the 1960 Annual Meeting in which a majority of the Divisions supported DDR, but others still actively opposed it. In addition, the number of Directors-at-Large was under study, since it too had been questioned. Up to that time, the Board of Directors consisted of approximately 60 individuals. It was thought that expanding it to 120 or more plus the Directors-at-Large would produce an unwieldy Board, and thrust more power on the executive committee. However, the committee recommended that this plan be submitted to the membership at the October Annual Meeting. The committee then met as a Reference Committee on October 25, 1961, and presented these recommendations.

Charles Ebersol recalls that at one of these meetings, which were held in a room at the Commodore Hotel on Forty-second Street in New York City, the "discussion was hot and heavy. We all cooled down when the sprinkler system unexpectedly let go."

"After discussion (which required seven pages of minutes)," Dr. Carlile noted, "the Reference Committee adopted a motion approving direct division representation in principle, with the recommendation that the president appoint a committee to work out the final details and report prior to June 1962."

"It was the lay leadership that carried on the fight over the organizational issue, as it had on United Way," Frank Wilcox recalls. "This was normal, as these issues were not primarily medical. The doctors were supportive and involved, but not to the degree that the laity were."

Wrote Dr. Carlile:

> Dr. Pendergrass chaired the committee again. It met December 1961 in Biloxi, Mississippi, where the preliminary report was developed that was presented to the Board meeting in January 1962. [Behind these bland words was a rancorous meeting, with both sides lined up to do battle. DDR was not quite as divisive as the United Way issue, but nearly led to a split in the Society.] The final proposal was presented June 1962 to the Board of Directors. This included a House of Delegates with proportional representation based on population with at least two delegates (one medical, one lay) from each Division. From these delegates, one Director from each Division would be nominated and be elected by the House of Delegates. There was no change in the number of Directors-at-Large. The regional meetings would be discontinued. This proposal was adopted at the meeting of members on October 24–25, 1962. This required a revision of the by-laws with the reorganization to become effective at the annual meeting in 1963.

Richard P. McGrail, the Society's former deputy executive vice-president, likens the expanded board, with one director from each division, to the United States Senate; and the House of Delegates, in which larger divisions have more members, to the U.S. House of Representatives. "It brought a greater representation of divisions on the board—it comes out to about two-thirds division-based directors, and about one-third directors-at-large. I think it has been very healthy because nobody feels that he is without a vote."

The National ACS board now consists of about 120 members; the total fluctuates in relation to the number of past officer-directors (who can be elected for three terms of two years each) and honorary life members (usually all past officer-directors are elected honorary life members after serving six years on the board).

As a result, the important work of the Society has to be relegated to fifty-six committees and subcommittees of the board, and a half-dozen work groups and task forces. Lane Adams explains:

> They all report to the board. So there isn't quite as much dialogue as there once was at board meetings. But the system works well. Everybody feels involved and participating, and that's the name of the game. Before, they felt something like taxation without representation. They were paying their sixty percent of revenues to National, but they felt they didn't have much voice in policy formulation. That's no longer the case.

Says Frank Wilcox, who participated vigorously in the major policy changes regarding United Way and direct division representation:

> We almost split apart on the issue of structure. We did split apart locally on the issue of finances and public education. But both judgments appear to have been wise, because of the results. The strength of the Society and its growth since those two steps were taken is proof. But they were risky at the time. They took courage, and a firm commitment to the principles involved: to independence, and to fair representation."

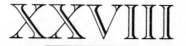

XXVIII

Cancer Becomes a National Priority: The National Cancer Acts

When I asked my husband for money for the American Cancer Society to do research, he said, "No, I'm not going to give you any money"—although he did. But he said, "The place to get the money is the federal government." And I said, "I don't know anything about the government." And he said, "There are unlimited funds. I'll show you how to get them."

—Mary Lasker

As Albert Lasker predicted, cancer research would require resources much greater than those of any private agency. The American Cancer Society has been a consistent leader in research. It organized the national extramural cancer-research program, which the government later supported. It could be innovative, move faster than the federal research agency, and inspire others to follow new paths in research. But basically its strength is in its volunteers and their programs, while the government has access to the large amounts of money needed to underwrite research projects too vast for private support— such as the search for anticancer drugs.

The federal government had been involved in intramural cancer research since the 1937 National Cancer Institute Act,

210

which boiled up spontaneously and nearly simultaneously out of the House of Representatives and the Senate. In 1936, in the House, Maury Maverick (D-Texas), spurred by a San Antonio constituent, Dr. Dudley Jackson, had introduced a bill to establish a national cancer institute. In the Senate, Senator Hugh Bone, (D-Washington) independently introduced a similar bill, and was able to get the signatures of all ninety-six U.S. senators in support. He also persuaded a Washington State representative, Warren Magnusson, to introduce the same bill in the House. The Bone-Magnusson bill superseded Maverick's.

Articles in *Fortune, Time,* and *Life* in support of the joint measure elicited heavy mail to Congress. The American Medical Association opposed the bill, its *Journal* warning that "the danger of putting the government in a dominant position in relation to medical research is apparent." The ASCC director, Dr. Clarence C. Little, came out for the legislation. In general, the ASCC position mirrored the activist attitude on the part of the public and legislators about the government's role in health. But, as illustrated by the AMA's statement, most physicians felt otherwise.

Dr. Little gained powerful support inside the White House by recruiting Mrs. Eleanor Roosevelt into the Women's Field Army. After joint House/Senate hearings in June, the Bone-Magnusson bill became law and the sum of $700,000 was appropriated for the National Cancer Institute's first budget, of which less than half was actually funded (President Franklin D. Roosevelt had asked for a million).

The Institute was a division of the Public Health Service, under the command of the surgeon general, Dr. Thomas Parran, who was at first opposed to the "categorical" disease approach to public health. Like most public-health authorities, he preferred an overall attack. But a decade later, Mary Lasker was able to involve Dr. Parran in going to Congress for another categorical disease institute: the National Heart Institute. The act establishing it was based on the National Cancer

Institute Act. There are now ten National Institutes of Health.

As soon as the National Cancer Institute was established, the national advisory cancer council called for in the enabling legislation was appointed, including two world-class scientists, James B. Conant chemist, and Arthur H. Compton, physicist, and three leading physician-investigators, James Ewing, Ludvig Hektoen, and Francis Carter Wood, as well as Dr. Little. They created a national program, part of which consisted of buying radium (9.5 grams for $200,000) and lending it to treatment centers. The council also created clinical and research fellowships, set up cooperation with state agencies, and organized intramural research and public education.

The NCI's budgets were extremely modest, rising to only $561,000 by 1945. World War II was not a time when the government could give much to long-term medical research. Besides, most of the brightest scientists and research-minded physicians were involved in the war effort.

It wasn't until after the war that the government role in cancer research picked up—thanks in large part to Albert Lasker's prescience. He counseled his wife to go to Washington, and she did. Although she had no experience in government, Mary Lasker spent the better part of nine months in 1945–46 in Washington, thus beginning a lifelong involvement in national politics as related to health research. She kept in close touch with the heads of committees responsible for research appropriations. She gave money to political campaigns in both parties. She had help and direction from the extremely savvy publicists Anna Rosenberg Hoffman and Emerson Foote, as well as from such medical leaders as Dr. Michael DeBakey, the famous heart surgeon, and Dr. Howard Rusk, the great innovator in physical rehabilitation.

In 1952 Albert Lasker died of cancer. That same year, Congressman John Fogarty introduced Colonel Luke Cornelius Quinn, USAF (ret.), to Mary Lasker. Colonel Quinn had been the air-force liaison with Congress since the end of World War II. Mary Lasker arranged for him to be the first Washington representative of the ACS. William Lewis, ACS chairman, and Dr. Sidney Farber of Boston Children's Hospital, a pioneer in treating childhood leukemia, decided that the only way to speed progress against cancer was to involve the government more deeply in funding research. They conceived the idea, their path eased by Colonel Quinn, of appearing as *amici curiae* when the National Cancer Institute presented its annual budget request before Congress.

Says Dr. Michael B. Shimkin of the University of California School of Medicine at San Diego, who worked at the National Cancer Institute from 1938 to 1963:

> The Lasker fortune could have established a research institution, along the format of the Rockefeller Institute for Medical Research. But Albert Lasker thought in bigger terms of involving the national treasury through appropriations. And the way to that goal was to organize a lobby for biomedical research allocations. . . . The Society represented a ready-made lobby group that already extended into the National Advisory Cancer Council of the National Cancer Institute.

Cancer evoked the same intensity of interest from senators and representatives as it did from the public. Legislators were always interested in progress reports from cancer experts. These were good reasons to vote funds for the NCI. Mary Lasker well understood this in her successful lobbying for research support.

Dr. Shimkin went on to say that

> Mary Lasker occupies and will be remembered for a commanding role in biomedical research in the United States. She followed the tactical plan laid out by her husband, not only for cancer but for mental and cardiac diseases, the three most prominent causes of disability and death. The plan involved a small, effective group of professional and governmental people at key points in the voluntary organizations, such as the American Cancer Society, in government, and well-placed money and

educational materials. . . . The latter included slick prints of the problem and its solution, to be placed on the desks of all congressmen and not simply mailed and thus forgotten. Generous support, then quite legal, was made available for election campaigns of a few well-selected converts, especially Lister Hill in the Senate and John E. Fogarty in the House. Memberships on councils that recommended the distribution of subsequent funds closed the circle. Direct access to the White House, and rewarding research scientists by prizes and statuettes of the Victory of Samothrace [the Lasker Foundation Awards] were useful reinforcements. . . . It was an effective extrapolation to its logical extremes of the advertising-mercantile culture of the United States, applied to goals considered worthy by the medical-scientific community.

Spurred by the effective lobbying of the ACS, the NCI budget began growing rapidly. In 1950 it totaled nearly $19 million; in 1960 it had risen to $91 million; and by 1970 to $190 million. Total NCI research grants were just under $100 million that year.

But progress against cancer was agonizingly slow, especially to Senator Ralph W. Yarborough (D-Texas), a disciple of Lister Hill. In the early 1960s Yarborough heard Dr. Randolph Lee Clark, director of the internationally esteemed M. D. Anderson Hospital and Tumor Institute in Houston, Texas, testify for the NCI research budget. Yarborough respected Dr. Clark, the more so because another member of the Clark family—well known among Texas educators—had inspired him to study law and to run for the Senate. The senator, who had lost several members of his family to cancer, asked Clark what would be needed to make a real breakthrough in curing the disease.

"It would take one billion dollars a year for ten years to find the answers for perhaps ninety percent of human cancers," Clark told the Senate Health Subcommittee. At the same time he said, "We can't use that kind of money now. We lack the facilities and the scientists to mount that level of attack."

Several years later, in 1969, Ralph Yarborough succeeded Lister Hill as head of the subcommittee. Mary Lasker, who had worked to get the job for Ted Kennedy, was disappointed, but not defeated. Her overriding purpose was to get the government behind an all-out effort to end cancer. Merely lobbying to increase the NCI's budget by increments wasn't doing it; legislation was needed. She would have to work with Yarborough. She began by suggesting he take on the job of getting a bill through Congress.

The senator, who was reputed to have a short attention span, listened. He recalled Dr. Clark's statement, and remembered how massive government efforts had built the first atomic bomb and put the first man on the moon. He agreed that the time was ripe for a similar endeavor to wipe out cancer. In March 1970 he introduced a resolution "supported by fifty-three of my colleagues in the Senate, calling for a completely new study of cancer, cancer research, and the causes and cure of the disease. The intent of this resolution is to make the conquest of cancer a national goal of the highest priority," according to a report to Congress.

A panel of twenty-six persons—thirteen eminent scientists and physicians and thirteen lay persons—was selected to do the study. The thirteen professionals were not only authorities in their fields, but several, like Drs. Mathilde Krim and William B. Hutchinson, had important political connections; and others, including Dr. Sidney Farber, were past or future ACS presidents. Mary Lasker arranged to have Democrats Emerson Foote, Anna Rosenberg Hoffman, and Lew Wasserman among the lay persons. She asked Laurance Rockefeller to help select some Republicans. Among them was Benno C. Schmidt, managing partner of the New York investment-banking firm of J. H. Whitney & Company, who was also a trustee (later chairman) of Memorial Sloan-Kettering Hospital. Schmidt and Farber became the panel's cochairmen. The Senate appropriated $250,000 for the investigation and report. Perhaps unique in the history of such enterprises, the committee spent only about 30 percent ($75,000) of the appropriation.

Chairman Schmidt submitted the report on November 25, 1970. Although 289 "members of the scientific community" had given oral or written testimony to the committee, itself a diverse group, and there were many divergent views, the report represented a consensus, Schmidt wrote in his letter of submittal. "The committee is unanimously of the view that the conquest of cancer is a realistic goal if an effective national program along the lines recommended in the report is promptly initiated and relentlessly pursued."

Congress anticipated the committee's consensus with one of their own. On July 15, 1970, several months before the committee report was finished, both houses passed a resolution stating that it was "the unanimous sense of the Congress that the conquest of cancer is a national crusade," and that the necessary funds should be appropriated.

The panel of consultants identified seventeen areas of cancer research that warranted "expanded and particularly vigorous exploration":

1. Epidemiology: Cancer might be clinically controlled (or prevented) by identifying genetic predisposition, immunological impairment, hormonal effects, or metabolic differences in different populations.

2. Chemical Carcinogenesis: Studying neoplastic changes in tissue culture should identify hazardous chemicals and how they create cancer. Most compounds that cause cancer are transformed into proximate carcinogens with certain common chemical characteristics and behaviors. Interfering with their metabolic effects might block carcinogenesis or reverse it.

3. Virology: Viruses were known to cause cancer in animals and people. In order to protect against viruses, medicine needed to know how a virus initiates

cancer, why it can rest for long periods without expressing cancer, how the body defends against oncogenesis, how the same virus may cause cancer or some other disease, how a virus can be detected through chemical reactions, and how viruses and chemicals may interact to form cancers.

4. Tumor Antigens: The differences between antigens from normal cells and specific tumor cells can lead to the tolerance or rejection of tumors. These might be exploited.

5. Cellular Immune Mechanisms: "Failure of cellular mechanisms to eradicate emerging tumor populations may be the final step before a tumor becomes established. . . ." There is evidence that some, if not all, cancer cells have surface antigens different from normal cells.

6. Humoral Immunity: One or more of five immunoglobulins, with perhaps other proteins in blood or lymphatic fluid, may create immunity that kills tumor cells or, conversely, protects these cells. They may hold an important key to immunity against cancer.

7. Immunoprophylaxis and Immunotherapy: Immune-enhancing agents have been demonstrated effective in some childhood leukemias and in preventing and treating cancer in experimental animals. Both needed more study, especially as to timing and specific stimulants of immunity.

8. Diagnosis: Cancerous tumors secret substances in blood known as markers. Some had been discovered that were quite specific for certain cancers—alpha-fetoprotein, for example, is a good marker for liver cancer. Identifying and detecting such markers would aid in earlier diagnosis, and determine the effectiveness of treatment.

9. Chemotherapy: About fifty chemicals had been

found effective against cancers. Used in various combinations and sequences, some are the treatment of choice against such cancers as Hodgkin's disease and acute lymphocytic leukemia. More and better anticancer drugs could cure more types of cancer.

10. Tumor-Cell Kinetics: Understanding the growth characteristics of tumor cells, which produce different substances at different phases of their growth, helps in selecting the proper chemotherapeutic agent(s), and in timing their use.

11. Sanctuary: Some tumor cells, far from a capillary or behind the blood/brain barrier, "may enjoy a pharmacological sanctuary where adequate drug concentrations cannot reach them or exert lethal effects." More knowledge of this phenomenon was needed.

12. New Drugs: More were needed to interfere with critical steps in cancer-cell biosynthesis and metabolism. Understanding differences between normal and malignant cells with regard to metabolism and enzyme secretion might lead to better drug design.

13. Radiotherapy: New radiation sources may avoid anoxia—lack of oxygen—in tumor tissues, a condition that makes many tumors insensitive to radiation. Radiosensitizing chemicals might also help make radiation treatments more effective.

14. Surgical Improvements: Surgery to remove precancerous lesions could prevent the development of invasive and metastatic cancer. Combinations of surgery, radiation, and drugs might eliminate residual cancer cells, thus assuring cure.

15. Fundamental Biological Studies: These might disclose changes in the genetic basis of life, DNA, and of RNA, which carries genetic messages, leading to cancer cure or prevention. Documentation was needed of the chemical differences between tumors, as well as their common links.

16. The Nature of Cell Surface: Little was known of the chemical or physical nature of this vital barrier, which affects the cell's antigenic properties, as well as its nutrition and drug intake. The cell surface also controls to some extent the ability of the cell to invade adjacent structures and to metastasize.

17. Biological Organization: In multicellular animals, cells communicate. Since one of the features of cancer is the loss of the normal architectural arrangement of cells, something must go wrong with their communication system. To learn what factors influence this, it would be helpful to elucidate the chemistry of growth-regulating chemicals so that analogues and antagonists might be formulated.

Senator Yarborough translated the panel's recommendations into a bill, which he introduced in December 1970. However, Yarborough had been defeated by Lloyd Bentsen in the Democratic primary in Texas the previous May and could not be reelected. Senator Edward M. Kennedy (D-Mass.) and Jacob K. Javits (R-N.Y.) took over the task of shepherding Yarborough's cancer bill through the Senate. In January 1971 they introduced S. 34—the Conquest of Cancer bill—into the Ninety-second Congress.

Elmer Bobst, a member of the panel of consultants, and a close personal friend of President Richard M. Nixon, began telling the president about the upcoming cancer report and advised the panel that he had urged Nixon to take an interest in cancer. He and Benno Schmidt made sure that the panel's report came to the White House soon after it was presented to the Senate. Schmidt, Laurance Rockefeller, and G. Keith Funston, former head of the New York Stock Exchange and a panel member, all wrote to Nixon about the report.

Mary Lasker had seen to it that the public got involved. In 1969 she had paid for full-page advertisements, written by Colonel Quinn, in a number of leading newspapers. They had been inspired by a book entitled *Cure for Cancer: A National Goal*, by Solomon Garb, M.D., in 1968. Mrs. Lasker was impressed by Garb's activist arguments for establishing this goal. The ads called on the president "to begin to end this curse. . . . Why don't we try to conquer cancer by America's 200th birthday?" In April 1971 she persuaded popular syndicated columnist Ann Landers to inform her millions of readers about cancer's dreadful toll and ask them to "become part of the mightiest offensive against a single disease in the history of our country" by writing to their state's U.S. senators at least a three-word message: "Vote for S. 34" (the Kennedy-Javits bill). Millions of letters poured into the Senate in support.

Schmidt and Mary Lasker suggested to Elmer Bobst in December 1970 that "it would be a wonderful idea" for Nixon to include the conquest of cancer in his State of the Union address in January 1971. Prompted by his chief of management and budget, George Shultz, his chief of staff for domestic affairs, John Erlichman, and a number of Republican businessmen who were perhaps inspired by Rockefeller, Bobst, Schmidt, and company, Nixon did include among his six goals in his State of the Union speech the following:

> I will ask for an appropriation of an extra $100 million to launch an intensive campaign to find a cure for cancer, and I will ask later for whatever additional funds can effectively be used. The time has come in America when the same kind of concentrated effort that split the atom and took man to the moon should be turned toward conquering this dread disease. Let us make a total national commitment to achieve the goal.

Later, the White House would introduce its own cancer bill in the Senate bearing Nixon's imprimatur: S. 1828.

There was disagreement over who should run the government's cancer crusade. The panel in its report had indicated dissatisfaction with the NCI's handling of cancer research and said that "the necessary administrative setup would not be easy to achieve within the federal government. . . . When the federal government has desired to give top priority to a major scientific project . . . it has on occasion, with considerable success, given the responsibility to an independent agency." The panel went on to recommend that the functions, personnel, programs, etc., of the NCI be transferred to a new National Cancer Authority, which "should be headed by an administrator appointed by the President with the advice and consent of the Senate, and he should report directly to the President and present his budgets and programs to the Congress."

After the Senate passed S. 1828, by a vote of seventy-nine to one (the one was Gaylord Nelson), the House of Representatives Subcommittee on Public Health and Environment (of the Committee on Interstate and Foreign Commerce) held hearings on making the conquest of cancer a national priority. Then joint House/Senate committee work finally created a bill that would pass both houses.

This sticky issue of who would be in charge of the cancer program was finally decided by compromise: The national cancer program would remain within the NCI, and a three-man panel would act as liaison between the president and the program director. There would be a separate budget for the NCI.

Satisfied with the achievement, and willing to relinquish credit, Javits and Kennedy withdrew S. 34 in favor of the nearly identical S.1828 from the White House. Congress finally passed this bill, credited to Richard M. Nixon, who signed it into law in January 1971 as the National Cancer Act of 1971. It was the first statute by any nation to make the conquest of cancer a national priority. Mr. Nixon has since said that it was the single most important contribution he made as president.

Funding followed political success. The NCI budget jumped from $233 million in 1971 to $379 million the following year, and rose to more than $1 billion by 1984.

Singling out cancer for special treatment created a good deal of envy among researchers in other fields, and among other Institutes of Health. The result was a spate of criticism against the idea of patterning the conquest of cancer on the model of a Manhattan Projct, or NASA. It was pointed out that while those organizations had had the necessary research base and needed only to make and test hardware, in cancer the research base was lacking.

Much of this criticism has since been muted by the advances made under the new cancer authority. Many of the seventeen fields of research identified by the panel have yielded substantial progress against cancer in the intervening years. In fact, it is generally agreed that more has been learned about the disease since 1971 than in all previous history.

The public attention focused on cancer by the legislative debate over the Cancer Act not only helped Congress justify funding cancer research, it also informed many people, whose quickest and most direct response was to give to and/or volunteer for the American Cancer Society.

During the 1970s the Society achieved the "impossible" goal of raising more than $1 billion from public contributions. This provided at least $300 million of additional ACS research support. It helped fund a number of new types of initiatives, such as the Research Development Program—enabling rapid funding of a new and promising field; and the Special (Five-Year) Institutional Grants to explore new and unanticipated needs in cancer cause and prevention. It is probably no exaggeration to attribute much of the exponential increase in cancer cures—from about one in three cases in the 1960s to one in two today—to the direct and indirect effects of the National Cancer Act of 1971. At current levels of incidence, this means saving about 100,000 additional American lives each year.

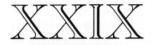

Public Issues

The American Cancer Society, many of whose directors have ties with major industries, places the emphasis on diagnosis and cures, rather than prevention. . . . the American Cancer Society has shown little interest in the environmental origins of cancer, many of which are in industrial processes and products.

from "Waging The Wrong War On Cancer," by Daniel S. Greenberg and Judith E. Randal, *The Washington Post*, May 1, 1977.

In 1969 the ACS hired McKinsey & Company to examine its management operations. At the end of their report, McKinsey offered unrelated comment—that cancer was becoming a matter of public concern and therefore a political issue—and they recommended establishing a Washington office.

The Society Washington representative Colonel Luke Quinn, had good connections in both houses of Congress. And the ACS had close relations with NCI—some ACS directors and staff served on NCI committees, and some NCI staff members participated in ACS medical and scientific meetings. This avoided overlap and duplication of activities. Many leading researchers and institutions received funding from both organizations; this was seen as useful, for it ensured research independence and served as a hedge against cutbacks in government budgets.

Alan Davis, who had been hired as science editor of the ACS, and whose main function had been to organize the annual science writers' seminars, was given the new responsibility of liaison between the executive vice-president of the ACS and the director of the NCI. But the Society did not open a Washington office. Davis, working out of New York City, began attending meetings of the National Cancer Advisory Council and, in his words, delineating "areas of dialogue regarding the interface between the private sector and public sector in cancer research and control."

He established good personal relations with Dr. Carl Baker, head of the NCI, who had the reputation of being outspoken. Alan Davis found him sympathetic and willing to cooperate on issues of mutual interest. The two organizations had parallel aims and, of course, ACS experts had supported NCI cancer-research budget requests before Congress for years. The 1971 Cancer Act had given the NCI an additional area of responsibility: cancer control.

Baker knew that the ACS was heavily involved in cancer control, but it would be something new for the NCI. "What is cancer control?" Baker asked Davis.

Davis suggested that Dr. Baker write to Lane Adams for a formal definition of the phrase and some guidelines. Adams turned Baker's letter over to Arthur Holleb, who defined the term. Cancer control, Holleb told Baker, is the application of the latest basic and clinical research findings to the diagnosis, cure, and rehabilitation of cancer patients. Thus, it is necessarily a community-based enterprise. This made it an obvious ACS priority, since the organization has volunteers and staff in nearly all of the nation's counties, cities, and towns. In 1971 the NCI had no such network, but it did have a greatly expanded budget, with $4 million earmarked for cancer control. Therefore, it was in the interests of cancer patients that the two organizations coordinate their efforts, each bringing its special strengths into the collaboration. Holleb also gave examples of the Society's cancer-control initiatives. One was the Breast Cancer Detection Demonstration Project (BCDDP) just then being organized. The Holleb letter was the first step in bringing the NCI into the BCDDP. The ACS had appropriated $1 million to study 12,000 women in twelve centers for two years. When the NCI decided to join in with ample government funds, the project expanded to take in 27 centers and 285,000 women for five years. Proving the accuracy of McKinsey's forecast, connections between the environment and health, particularly cancer, had begun worrying the public. These can be traced back to the early 1960s, when Swedish scientists identified several severe ecological emergencies that cried out for action: Acid rain was killing forests and destroying rivers and lakes all around the northern hemisphere; oil spills and sewage were turning seas such as the Baltic and Mediterranean, and long stretches of many continental coastlines, into disaster areas; heavy metals and DDT were accumulating in fish and shellfish from the Atlantic to the China Sea and decimating bird populations that fed on marine organisms.

Some of these problems were first dramatized in 1962 by Rachel Carson in her book *Silent Spring*. This was followed by books and articles by other popular writers. The sudden revelation of previously unknown hazards lurking beneath the seas and polluting the air, threatening health and life almost everywhere, shocked the public. Suddenly, millions of people became apprehensive and mistrustful of their governments' efforts to protect them, and antagonistic toward private industry and commerce. Their level of apprehension and distrust rose, especially in the United States, during the Vietnam War. This conflict seriously eroded Americans' faith in the commitment of government and of private enterprise to protect the environment, especially when massive amounts of toxic defoliants and herbicides were dumped indiscriminately on American soldiers, Vietnamese and wildlife, as well as on trees and plants.

When the war ended, a great residue of public concern and suspicion focused on possible links between environmental pollution and cancer. This led to legislative action like the

Toxic Substances Control Act of 1976. Until then the ACS had never taken an active position on an entire piece of legislation except the Cancer Acts; it had been Society policy to comment only on those aspects of bills that related to cancer.

To quote from an ACS memorandum: "The Toxic Substances Control Act of 1976 created considerable debate among consumerists, environmentalists, business, industry and government. The Society was under considerable pressure to 'endorse' [the bill], and one newspaper column characterized the Society as 'cowardly' for not doing this." However, the ACS had decided not to endorse the bill for two reasons: First, it was mainly a regulatory statute, and the ACS felt that its own expertise was not in regulation; and second, although "it was a broad piece of legislation, [it] made no reference to controlling the most toxic of substances known to cause cancer: tobacco and tobacco products."

However, said Alan Davis, the Society put forward "a strong statement about the potential dangers of toxic substances, requested a congressional review and urged the Congress to act if it determined that real problems existed."

As Davis has noted, when Congress passed the Toxic Substances Act, "there was some concern that President Ford might veto it." Since the Society was on record as supporting any law in this area that Congress might enact, its president, Dr. Benjamin F. Byrd, Jr., wrote to Ford: "speaking for the 2.5 million volunteers of the American Cancer Society, I commend this legislation to you, and urge that you sign it into law."

President Ford did sign the bill. But the ACS, which had been castigated for not supporting it during the legislative process, was now criticized for trying to head off the veto. Some of the bill's supporters claimed that the Cancer Society was trying to take credit for it.

This was an example of the new political problems the ACS and other institutions had begun to face. It was also a reflection of the suspicion with which all sorts of institutions were regarded by activist groups and the news media. This had begun with the Watergate scandal, which highlighted the Woodward/Bernstein brand of investigative journalism. Proved so effective (and rewarding) in uncovering a political cover-up, it became the model for many reporters in other fields. They began taking a much more truculent, adversarial approach not only toward public officials but toward all large organizations, whether for-profit corporations or eleemosynary groups like the American Cancer Society supposedly devoted to the public weal.

As Deep Throat had fed politically explosive questions and leads to Woodward and Bernstein, many scientists and medical researchers raised questions about the cancer field. These people opposed the National Cancer Act as giving special status and budget increases to cancer research and control at the expense, they claimed, of other biomedical research and disease control. They called proponents of the Cancer Act "the cancer establishment" and drew analogies between the fight against cancer and the Vietnam War ("the body count") to the new breed of reporters. Unfortunately, many of the latter were uninstructed in science and medicine. Impressed with the credentials of Cancer Act critics they were unequipped to evaluate their criticism and unaccustomed to doing the kind of research needed to make judicious assessments. The critics' own agendas were often unexamined; their statements appeared intact in the media.

And there were other, more malevolent sources of attack on the cancer program and the American Cancer Society. Disaffected researchers, and promoters of unproved cancer remedies that the Society had consistently exposed, were suddenly given public credence in the media. The media also frequently quoted perennial critics of the ACS, such as Dr. Bailar of the NCI, Dr. Irwin Bross of Roswell Park Memorial Institute, and Samuel Epstein, author of a book called *The Politics of Cancer*.

Thus, almost overnight the American Cancer Society was the target of public attacks by what appeared to be a sudden confluence of interest between cancer quacks, fringe health groups, and some respected researchers.

The major points of censure were summed up in a long article in the *Washington Post* by Daniel S. Greenberg and Judith E. Randal, titled "Waging the Wrong War Against Cancer." These reporters had long experience in reporting science and medicine, and of course the newspaper had national standing as an exposer of corruption in high places, so their detailed critique had to be taken seriously.

Its central theses were that the ACS "places the emphasis on diagnosis and cures, rather than prevention," and that it "has shown little interest in the environmental origins of cancer, many of which are in industrial processes and products." The Society's alleged disinterest in environmental carcinogens was attributed by the authors to powerful industrial and banking interests on its board of directors.

In a short rebuttal printed by the *Post* twelve days after the Greenberg/Randal article, Society president Dr. R. Lee Clark and Frank J. Rauscher, senior vice-president for research, made the following points:

• "As an organization started and directed by volunteers to fight cancer, it is obviously our first priority to do everything we can to reduce [cancer's] intolerable toll."

• Although environmental sources probably account for between 50 and 90 percent of all cancers, these sources are much more far-ranging than Greenberg and Randal assumed. Cigarette smoking is implicated in about 30 percent of all cancer deaths. An unknown number may be related to diet. "Between 1 and 2 percent [of cancers] occur because of intense exposure to carcinogens in the workplace; an estimated 3 percent are related to long-term exposure in the general environment; perhaps 5 percent are related to the use of medications in controlling deadly human diseases," Clark and Rauscher wrote.

• "The American Cancer Society has led the fight against known carcinogens in the environment," starting with smoking, then "helping to identify asbestos and polyvinyl chloride as carcinogenic dangers to workers," and working with producers, processors, and trade unions to control these substances. The Society had also identified cancer risks among aniline-dye and rubber workers, woodworkers, nickel miners, uranium miners, and roofers.

• Thus, the Society's record against carcinogens in the environment is long-standing, and has overlooked no known hazard. The *Post*'s imputation that the Society's exposure of workplace carcinogens was limited or suppressed by "bankers and industrialists" on the board was thus palpably without foundation. Had the authors bothered to check, they would have found no industrialists on the ACS board, and only a single representative of a major bank. Less than 3 percent of ACS income came from corporate gifts.

The Greenberg/Randal piece also charged that "powerful and magnetic" personalities at the ACS were controlling NCI; this was denied by both organizations. But it was a fact that people from both organizations served on each other's committees.

Six weeks after the piece appeared, the subcommittee of the Committee on Government Operations of the House of Representatives held hearings under chairman L. H. Fountain of North Carolina—a state where tobacco is the leading cash crop—about the "progress and administration" of the National Cancer Program. The approach of the congressmen may be judged from the opening statement of the leading minority member, John W. Wydler of New York. Mr. Wydler asked, "Are we spending our money as effectively as we should?" He questioned whether it ought to go into basic research, or prevention, or focus on treatment and cure. "I am disturbed," he said, "when I hear that the quality of research supported by federal moneys is not as good as it should be.

. . . Knowing that the war on cancer is now a multimillion-dollar business, I wonder about the potential conflicts of interest between those who grant the money and those who do the research."

Much was made of the fact that three staff members of NCI, Drs. Frank Rauscher, Guy R. Newell, Jr., and R. A. Tjalma had been paid a few hundred dollars' worth of travel and hotel expenses by the ACS to attend ACS meetings. (In one case the money came from a special gift to the ACS earmarked for this purpose.)

While no improprieties were evidenced, in order to eliminate even the appearance of influence by one organization in the other, the ACS Board of Directors voted in 1977 to drop all dual responsibilities and to refuse any joint funding with the NCI of projects such as the BCDDP in the future. A few projects had to be phased out slowly; five years was set as the outside limit. Cooperation was permitted between the ACS and government agencies, but no shared funding. These policies have been followed ever since. The ACS still testifies for the NCI's budget requests, and cooperates enthusiastically with NCI on projects of mutual interest, but there is total separation of personnel and budgets. "The relationship is close, but no touching," says Alan Davis.

The fact that most cancers are probably "caused by the environment" had first been disseminated by the Society more than ten years before the *Post* article, but had been misunderstood almost as often as it was discussed by journalists and the public. Very few nonprofessionals knew that the concept was based on comparisons of the wide differences in incidence of similar tumors in different countries (see chapter XX). Most people—even many seasoned medical journalists like Greenberg and Randal—assumed that environmental causation meant air and water pollution by industrial chemicals; whereas Dr. John Higginson, who had created the concept, had specified a wide range of possible etiologies, including personal behavior and habits.

The fear of cancer is probably the most powerful force behind the environmental movement, yet despite attacks on the Society, the public continued to regard it as the leading authority on cancer. People came to the organization for opinions regarding environmental carcinogens, and consumer groups pressured the ACS for statements and action.

At the time, the Society had no machinery for responding to these new demands. With the exception of smoking and a handful of industrial carcinogenic compounds mentioned earlier, and cancers caused by overexposure to sunlight and ionizing radiation, the ACS had been involved mainly in questions of research, diagnosis, treatment, and rehabilitation. An implicit policy had grown up of dealing with public issues involving cancer only on the basis of science and medicine. There had always been time to consider issues carefully before taking positions. But now the ACS was being importuned by the media and by the public for immediate answers to unanticipated, worrisome new questions. So many substances suddenly were suspected of causing cancer that the expression "carcinogen of the week" came into currency.

Perhaps the gravest of these, from the Society's point of view, was saccharin. This substance, discovered in 1879, had been first employed as a no-calorie sweetener in canned goods in the early 1900s, had been used by many millions of people as a sugar substitute during the two world wars, and had been a mainstay of diabetic diets for at least fifty years. In 1972 a long-term U.S. study of rats indicated that saccharin was a cause of animal bladder cancer. Two generations of rats had been fed a lifetime diet of which 5 percent consisted of saccharin. This was an enormous proportion of the sweetener, equivalent to an average person's drinking about 1,500 saccharin-sweetened sodas every day for a full lifetime. In the second generation, the *male rats only* developed many more bladder tumors than the "control" rats (those not fed saccharin). When a similar Canadian study several years later confirmed the effect, the U.S. Food and Drug Administration published its intention of removing saccharin from the market. It had no choice in the matter under the law; the Delaney clause in the Food and Drug Act states that if a food additive is found to cause cancer in animals, it must be banned in this country.

However, since saccharin was the only no caloric sweetener in the U.S. market, there was an immediate outcry from diabetics and dieters. Literally millions of letters poured into Congress, and the ACS was forced to issue a statement. If the Society chose to rely on the FDA, saccharin had to be considered carcinogenic. But they knew that the FDA had no options in the matter, and they were aware of doubts as to whether animal tests were predictive of human cancer. There were other health issues as well: the value of a no-calorie sweetener in helping to control diabetes and obesity—the latter associated with an increased risk of cancer as well as diabetes, heart and circulatory disease.

In March 1977 an ad hoc group of ACS executives, including Dr. Arthur Holleb and Dr. Frank Rauscher, got together to draw up a statement, which they checked via telephone with Thomas Ulmer, the ACS chairman, who lived in Jacksonville, Florida, and Dr. R. Lee Clark, president, in Houston, Texas. The underlying fact was that there was no scientific or medical certainty regarding saccharin's safety or risk for human beings. The rat studies had indicated risk; but Dr. Guy R. Newell, Jr., acting head of the National Cancer Institute, told Congress, which was considering a moratorium on the FDA's ban of saccharin, "We have no evidence that saccharin causes cancer in humans."

Many scientists were dubious about the dangers of saccharin. It was unlikely that a substance so widely used for so many years would suddenly turn out to be a powerful human carcinogen. Besides, it did not fit the general picture of a carcinogen: It did not affect DNA, and it was rapidly excreted intact (not metabolized) by the kidneys. Dr. Alexander Schmidt, the previous FDA commissioner, urged that Congress permit the sweetener to stay on the market by setting a "level of tolerable risk" under which "a weak carcinogen might be judged safe as a tabletop sweetener, if properly labeled."

The ACS committee weighed all the evidence and came up with a position paper on March 25, 1977. It did not accept that saccharin was an immediate, serious hazard to health. The committee pointed out that the FDA was mandated to act under the Delaney Amendment, and that the principle of that amendment was "basically sound." However, said the committee,

> as a major national voluntary health agency, the ACS is vitally concerned with the general health and well-being of the public. Saccharin is of great value in dietetic foods used to help control diabetes and obesity, which afflict tens of millions of Americans and pose more immediate dangers than the possible carcinogenicity of saccharin. Banning saccharin may cause great harm to many citizens while protecting a theoretical few.
>
> All evidence for and against saccharin should be further studied by independent scientists so that a course of action could be determined which would be of greatest benefit to the public. . . .
>
> Saccharin requires a special review by the Congress to determine if it should be exempt from the Delaney Amendment.

The Society was castigated by consumer groups for refusing to protect the public. There were innuendos that the ACS had been pressured by the soft-drink industry to downplay saccharin's risk. The ACS statement came out just before its 1977 Science Writers' Seminar; at the seminar it was used as a club by a number of leading journalists to beat the ACS. A highly respected ACS-funded scientist and Nobel laureate, Dr. David Baltimore, made common cause with the journalists and criticized the ACS leadership for not supporting the FDA's ban.

Much of this censure found its way into print and other media, but the Society stuck to its position. Congress did place a moratorium on the FDA's ban of saccharin, and has since renewed the moratorium five times—the latest for two years, until April 1987. And in 1978 Dr. Baltimore told Alan Davis that the ACS had been right after all not to panic in the face of pressure. There is still, nine years later, no evidence of human cancer caused by saccharin. At least twenty studies among many thousands of people, a number of them diabetics who consumed large quantities of saccharin for years or decades, have shown no increase in bladder cancer among saccharin users as compared with nonusers.

A more recent ACS statement urges caution and moderation in the use of artificial sweeteners (there is a second synthetic sweetener on the U.S. market at this time—aspartame), especially by children and pregnant women.

After saccharin, it was likely that more unsuspected environmental carcinogens, or supposed carcinogens, would surface. And it was clear that the ACS could not depend on its machinery to anticipate or deal with these problems.

Lane Adams called in Arthur D. Little & Company for advice, and they worked out a system for responding to such questions.

At the annual meeting in November 1977, the ACS Board of Directors voted to establish a new committee to deal with public issues. There would be two cochairmen—one medical and one lay—and "at least two-thirds of the committee shall be members of the Board of Directors of the Society." The new committee would be "responsible for advising on legislative and regulatory agency matters relating to cancer research or control . . . including but not limited to formulating policies and positions on legislative and regulatory matters that may affect the cancer patient and his family."

The Public Issues Committee, which included several well-known people who were not ACS board members, came into being in February 1978. Cochairmen were Dr. Benjamin F. Byrd, Jr., former president of the ACS, and Charles Ebersol, former ACS chairman.

The committee set up a "fast track" group, an executive committee of about a half-dozen people to deal with any urgent matters. This consisted of Dr. Byrd; Mr. Ebersol; Dr. R. Lee Clark; the Hon. Joseph Young, a longtime ACS volunteer who was a federal judge; and Dr. Harry Woolf, head of the Institute of Advanced Studies at Princeton, New Jersey.

However, the executive committee was created only for emergencies. Instead of waiting for environmental issues to develop, the Society set out to prospect for them so that the whole Public Issues Committee could have time to investigate and formulate reasoned positions in advance of crises. One of its most valuable members was Dr. Irving Selikoff of Mount Sinai Medical Center in New York City, an internationally known authority on carcinogens in the environment. Later, under a new form of research grant, the ACS contracted with Dr. Selikoff and his staff to alert them to possibly troublesome substances before they became matters of immediate public concern. Dr. Selikoff, the first researcher to concentrate on the cancers and other diseases caused by asbestos, was joined by Dr. Cuyler Hammond after the latter retired from the ACS. Hammond was also knowledgeable about industrial compounds linked to disease. The two investigators were in the best position to advise the ACS of any newly identified substances that might cause cancer in animals or humans. And they had files of information, and necessary expertise, to help supply answers to the Public Issues Committee.

Since 1978 the Public Issues Committee has issued opinions on about twenty different subjects, including hair dyes; 1,3-butadiene; benzene; formaldehyde; mass chest-X-ray screening; nutrition; cancer insurance; the use of heroin and marijuana for relieving the pain of cancer; nuclear energy; and a number of others. These statements are updated as new, pertinent information is received. Widely published and distributed, they are readily available from the American Cancer Society.

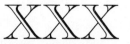

The Record

Ultimately an organizaiton, no matter how well intentioned, voluntary or not, for-profit or eleemosynary, has to be judged by its accomplishments. How close has the American Cancer Society come to its stated goal: "the control and eradication of cancer"?

In the following categories the Society is partly or largely responsible for progress:

CURE

When the American Society for the Control of Cancer started in 1913, there was no cure rate for any form of cancer. When the Society was reorganized in 1945, the cure rate for all cancers in the United States was estimated at one out of five cases. Today, in the United States, the survival rate is estimated at about 50 percent in all serious cancers (omitting the nearly 100 percent curable basal-cell skin cancers and *in situ* cancers of the cervix).

EDUCATION

The single most important factor in curing cancer is finding and treating it early. This required changing the public's concept of cancer as a kind of social disease that was invariably fatal into a malady that could be openly discussed, and could be cured. It also required educating the medical profession to the latest advances in diagnosis and therapy, and transforming the basic approach of therapeutic nihilism to one of aggressive activism. The importance of these changes in attitude and behavior cannot be overestimated; that they were mainly set in motion by the American Cancer Society is indisputable.

RESEARCH

When the ACS was reorganized in 1945, there was no national cancer-research program worthy of the name. Today, U.S. cancer research is the largest and most productive area of biomedical research in the world. It is the source of the great advances in cancer diagnosis, treatment, and cure. The ACS blazed the path by investing nearly $900 million dollars in research. And it helped to educate the Congress to create the National Cancer Acts of 1937 and 1971. The latter made the conquest of cancer a priority of government for the first time anywhere in the world. It is responsible for much of the great progress against cancer since its passage. Cancer research and professional education are responsible for progress made in the following four categories: chemotherapy, radiotherapy, surgery, and the increase in comprehensive cancer centers.

CHEMOTHERAPY

In 1945 no safe and effective drugs existed with which to cure cancer. Today, there are about fifty useful anticancer medications; they are the treatment of choice for about twenty kinds of cancer, and in about nine types they can cure the great majority of cases. An estimated 50,000 people are cured of cancer each year in the United States by or with anticancer drugs. As adjurant therapy with other treatments cancer drugs are adding to survival as well.

RADIOTHERAPY

Forty years ago the general consensus of patients and doctors about radiotherapy was that using it meant there was no hope for the patient. It was mainly employed as palliation. Today, radiation therapy is responsible for about one-third of 326,000 cancer cures that are being effected—about 100,000 cases per year in the United States. In Hodgkin's disease and cancers of the breast, cervix, larynx, prostate, uterus, bladder, testicle, tongue, and floor of the mouth, results of radio therapy are at least comparable to those of surgery. There have also been great advances in the use of radiation to diagnose cancer and other diseases.

SURGERY

Still the leading method of treating cancer, surgery has become ever more effective and less mutilating. Alone, or combined with radiotherapy and/or chemotherapy, it is responsible for about half of the cancer cures now being effected—about 175,000 cases each year in the United States.

CANCER SPECIALISTS

While there have been doctors expert in cancer for decades, there were no "oncologists"—full-time cancer specialists—until the last twenty years. The prognosis for cancer patients used to be generally so poor that no doctor could devote his entire practice to the disease; morale would crack when the great majority of patients were almost certain to die.

Today, this is no longer the case. There are literally thousands of medical specialists who treat nothing but cancer throughout their careers: medical oncologists, surgical oncologists, radiation oncologists, as well as oncological nurses and paramedical personnel. Thus, today's cancer patients can be assured of the latest in diagnosis, therapy, and rehabilitation.

CANCER CENTERS

It was long known by experts that the comprehensive cancer centers, which focused the newest in research, training, equipment, technology, and expertise entirely on cancer, achieved a higher cure rate of difficult cancers than did other hospitals. When the American Cancer Society began, there were only three such centers in the United States: M. D. Anderson in Houston, Memorial Sloan-Kettering in New York City, and Roswell Park in Buffalo. Today, there are twenty-two comprehensive cancer centers strategically located throughout the country to be within reach of all cancer patients who need their specialized services—estimated to be about 15 percent of the total cancer case load. These are one result of the 1971 National Cancer Act. For most cancer patients, community hospitals now have sufficient expertise and equipment to give adequate care.

PREVENTION

The role played by the ACS in revealing the causative role of smoking in lung and other cancers, and its many programs to educate the public and medical profession, to keep youngsters from starting to smoke, and help smokers quit, add up to an enormous saving of life and improvement in health. The ACS has also for years attempted to protect the public from overexposure to sunlight, the major cause of skin cancer, including the dangerous melanoma. And it has been in the vanguard of identifying other carcinogens in the environment.

This is a short balance sheet of some major accomplishments. The bottom line is lives saved. There are 5 million Americans alive today who have had cancer. Three million have survived for five years since diagnosis. Most of these can be considered cured. The fifteen pioneers who founded the American Society for the Control of Cancer appear to have succeeded beyond their wildest imaginings. And the ultimate goal of wiping out cancer as a threat to human beings is now in sight.

Appendixes

Appendix A

Organizational Background of the American Society for the Control of Cancer

(From Mefford R. Runyon, "The American Cancer Society: A Profile." Paper read at the Biltmore Hotel, New York, N.Y., October 29, 1959.)

A.M.A. AND GYNECOLOGISTS APPOINT CANCER COMMITTEES

In 1905, at a meeting of the American Medical Association, Dr. Lewis McMurtry, President, proposed a committee to prepare a report on cancer mortality. This committee recommended:

1. education of physicians, and
2. education of the public, especially of women.

In May 1912, at a meeting of the American Gynecological Society in Baltimore, papers were presented by a number of doctors, including Dr. Howard C. Taylor, Sr., Dr. Thomas S. Cullen and Dr. Reuben Peterson, on Radical Abdominal Operation for Cancer of the Cervix. These papers made such an impression that it was decided a committee should be appointed to collect facts on this form of cancer and work out a plan of action to be presented at the next A.G.S. meeting.

243

A MEETING OF MEDICAL AND LAY LEADERS

In March 1913, this committee met with Dr. Clement Cleveland, an outstanding New York gynecologist, and requested that he appoint a committee of laymen and doctors to aid in the establishment of a national cancer society. The following week, a meeting of medical and lay leaders was held at Dr. Cleveland's home in New York City. Mrs. Robert G. Mead, Dr. Cleveland's daughter, always an inspired leader in the work, was present. It happened that all of the laymen who attended this meeting were residents of New York City. They decided not to form a permanent organization at that time, but merely to indicate to the American Gynecological Society the group's willingness to cooperate in such an undertaking. This seemed wise as someone observed, "We are always a little shy of anything that starts in New York," and it was decided that New York should be kept in the background.

A second meeting was held on April 22nd, 1913, again at Dr. Cleveland's home. Dr. Frederick L. Hoffman, statistician of the Prudential Life Insurance Company, was in attendance and stressed the increasing cancer mortality rate. Dr. Joseph L. Bryant suggested that a resolution be adopted to form an organization "for the purpose of putting before the public the necessity of taking steps to reduce the number of deaths from cancer."

THE SOCIETY IS BORN

The 38th Annual Convention of the American Gynecological Society was held in Washington the first week of May 1913. The Congress of American Physicians and Surgeons met at the same time. The entire second day of the Convention was devoted to the subject of cancer control. Dr. Hoffman again warned, "I am absolutely convinced that the cancer death rate is increasing and the larger recorded mortality is not primarily due to improved medical diagnosis and more accurate methods of death certification." He concluded his address with ten recommendations, one of which was for the organization of an American Society "for the study and prevention of cancer, primarily for the purpose of educating the public at large in the absolute necessity of operative treatment at the earliest indication of cancerous growth."

It is significant that cancer research was not mentioned as one of the functions of the proposed Society.

A meeting of ten doctors and five laymen at the Harvard Club followed on May 22nd, at which the Society was formally created. (See reference note for Chapter III for their names.) It was the culmination of lengthy reports, detailed studies and many conferences. The American Medical Association, the Congress of American Physicians and Surgeons, the American Gynecological Society, the Clinical Congress of Surgeons of North America, insurance companies, interested laymen and laywomen were all involved. Thus the Society at its birth could claim distinguished sponsorship.

The resolution adopted on May 22, 1913, was as follows:

"Resolved, that we form a Society for the following purposes: to disseminate knowledge concerning the symptoms, treatment and prevention of cancer; to investigate conditions under which cancer is found; and to compile statistics in regard thereto."

Two weeks later they named the infant organization THE AMERICAN SOCIETY FOR THE CONTROL OF CANCER.

Appendix B
Recommendations for an American Society for the Control of Cancer

(From Dr. Frederick L. Hoffman, in an address to the American Gynecological Society, May 7, 1913.)

1. The organization of an American Soiciety for the study and prevention of cancer, primarily for the purpose of educating the public at large in the absolute necessity of operative treatment at the earliest indication of cancerous growths.
2. A thorough investigaiton into the geographical distribution of cancer throughout the Western Hemisphere but with special reference to localities and sections which persistently show a very high or a very low rate of cancer mortality.
3. A thoroughly qualified medical and statistical investigation into the cancer experience data of general and cancer hospitals for a period of sufficient length to determine the precise results of medical and surgical treatment, with a due regard to the after-lifetime, possible recurrence, or subsequent death of patients discharged as cured or materially improved.
4. A nation-wide agitation for a material improvement and required completeness of the official returns of deaths from cancer, with a due regard to the organs or parts

affected, for the purpose of reducing the number and proportion of unclassified or ill-defined cancers to the lowest possible minimum.

5. The Division of Vital Statistics of the Census as well as all State and municipal boards of health in charge of the registration, tabulation and analysis of vital statistics should be urged to redistribute the deaths occurring in institutions according to the permanent or regular residence of the deceased. Only by means of such a correction can the true local incidence of cancer be established, as has been shown with admirable clearness by the investigations of Green, of Edinburgh.

6. A thoroughly scientific investigation, through the cooperation of the Census Office, the Bureau of Labor, the Bureau of Mines, Life Insurance Companies, etc., should be made into the occupational incidence of cancer, with regard to which there are strong reasons for believing that a wealth of useful information can be brought to light which is at present unavailable.

7. Since an erroneous diet is a probable causative factor in cancer occurrence, the nutrition of cancerous patients should be investigated in conformity with the strictly scientific and conclusive methods of Professors Atwater and Chitttenden.

8. As an aid in the scientific study of cancer, and as a possible means of bringing about a more intelligent public understanding of the accepted facts of cancer occurrence, its nature and probable cure, the disease should be made reportable to the Board of Health in the same manner as other diseases which are recognized menaces to public health and welfare.

9. As a further aid, the Department of Agriculture should be requested to make a thorough study of the occurrence of cancer among domestic animals and plants known, or suspected, to be subject thereto, and such an investigation should as far as practicable, be coordinated to the work of the Bureau of Soils.

10. The immediate preparation and widest distribution of a concise outline of accepted cancer facts, showing the disease in all cases to be of local origin, that the chief danger to the patient lies in the tendency toward a rapid extension of cancerous growths, that the only certain remedy known to science is the complete surgical removal of the affected parts at the earliest possible indication of the disease, and that when this is done the outlook for a cure in the accepted meaning of the term is decidedly hopeful, but that to the contrary delay and neglect or refusal to submit to operative treatment are practically certain to result fatally within a comparatively short period of time.

Appendix C
List of American Cancer Society Presidents

Prepared by the ACS Medical Library

1913–1919	Mr. George C. Clark
1919–1922	Charles A. Powers, MD
1922–1930	Howard C. Taylor, MD
1930–1932	Jonathan M. Wainwright, MD
1932–1934	George H. Bigelow, MD
1934–1936	Burton T. Simpson, MD
1936–1937	Robert B. Greenough, MD
1937–1938	Frederick F. Russell, MD
1938–1942	John J. Morton, Jr., MD
1942–1944	Herman C. Pitts, MD
1944–1947	Frank Adair, MD
1947–1948	Edwin P. Lehman, MD
1948–1949	C.C. Nesselrode, MD
1949–1950	Alton Ochsner, MD
1950–1951	Guy Aud, MD
1951–1952	Charles C. Lund, MD
1952–1953	Harry M. Nelson, MD
1953–1954	Alfred M. Popma, MD
1954–1955	Howard C. Taylor, Jr., MD
1955–1956	C.V. Brindley, MD
1956–1957	David A. Wood, MD
1957–1958	Lowell T. Coggeshall, MD
1958–1959	Eugene Pendergrass, MD
1959–1960	Warren Cole, MD

1960–1961	John W. Cline, MD
1961–1962	Thomas Carlile, MD
1962–1963	I.S. Ravdin, MD
1963–1964	Wendell G. Scott, MD
1964–1965	Murray M. Copeland, MD
1965–1966	Leonard W. Larson, MD
1966–1967	Ashbel C. Williams, MD
1967–1968	Roger A. Harvey, MD
1968–1969	Sidney A. Farber, MD
1969–1970	Jonathan E. Rhoads, MD, D.Sc.
1970–1971	H. Melvin Pollard, MD
1971–1972	A. Hamblin Letton, MD
1972–1973	Arthur G. James, MD
1973–1974	Justin J. Stein, MD
1974–1975	George P. Rosemond, MD
1975–1976	Benjamin F. Byrd, Jr., MD
1976–1977	R(andolph) Lee Clark, MD
1977–1978	R. Wayne Rundles, MD
1978–1979	La Salle D. Leffall, Jr., MD
1979–1980	Saul B. Gusberg, MD
1980–1981	Edward F. Scanlon, MD
1981–1982	Robert V.P. Hutter, MD
1982–1983	Willis J. Taylor, MD
1983–1984	Gerald P. Murphy, MD, D.Sc.
1984–1985	Robert J. McKenna, MD
1985–1986	Charles A. Le Maistre, MD
1986–1987	Virgil Loeb, Jr., MD

Appendix D
List of American Cancer Society Chairmen of the Board of Directors

Prepared by the ACS Medical Library

1937–3/42	Edwin B. Wilson, Ph.D., LL.D.
4/42–3/44	John J. Morton, Jr., MD
4/44–4/45	Herman C. Pitts, MD
5/45–5/46	Eric A. Johnston
6/46–3/48	Eric A. Johnston (Honorary)
6/46–1947	Ted R. Gamble
1948–1949	Eric A. Johnston (Chairman)
1949–1950	Eric A. Johnston (Honorary)
1949–1955	Elmer H. Bobst (Honorary)
1949–1952	William C. Donovan
1952/53–1959	Gov. Walter J. Kohler
1955–1956	James S. Adams (Honorary Chairman)
1959–1962	Rutherford B. Ellis
1957–to date	Mrs. Albert D. Lasker (Honorary Chairman)
1962–1966	Francis J. Wilcox
1966–1967	Travis T. Wallace
1967–1971	William B. Lewis
1971–1973	Charles R. Ebersol
1973–1975	Winston Armin Willig
1975–1977	Thomas P. Ulmer

1977–1980	Hon. Joseph H. Young
1980–1982	Allan K. Jonas
1982–1985	G. Robert Gadberry
1985–1986	Don Elliot Heald

Notes and
References

Notes and References

Asterisked notes are the author's comments on the main text. Other notes are bibliographical references.

CHAPTER I
Halfway to Victory

page   *3*   Relative survival rate of U.S. cancer patients: *1985 Cancer Facts & Figures* (New York: American Cancer Society, Inc., 1985), p. 3.

CHAPTER II
Cancer Risk

page   *9*   Estimated ratio of babies who will develop cancer: News Release, American Cancer Society, Inc., Feb. 14, 1985.

page   *10*   "Carcinogenesis": U.S. Congress. Senate. *Report of the National Panel of Consultants on the Conquest of Cancer.* 92d Cong., 1st sess. Senate Doc. 92-9 (Washington, D.C.: U.S. Government Printing Office, 1971), p. 69.

page   *13*   "I had an interview with the Board of Guardians. . . .": Quoted in L. Clendening, *Source Book of Medical History* (New York: Hoeber, 1942), pp. 469–70.

page   *14*   Scrotal cancer in chimney sweeps: P. Pott, *Chirurgical Observations Relative to the Cataract, the Polypus of the Nose, the Cancer of the Scrotum, the Different Kinds of Rupture, and the Mortification of the Toes and Feet* (London: Hawes, Clarke & Colling, 1775).

CHAPTER III
Organizing the Attack

page   *15*   "In no other does the patient . . .": C. S. Cameron, *The Truth About Cancer* (Englewood Cliffs, N.J.: Prentice-Hall, 1956), pp. 8–9.

page *15* The American Society for the Control of Cancer was founded on May 22, 1913 at the Harvard Club in New York City. The founders were ten physicians and five laymen: Dr. James Ewing of the Association of Pathologists and Bacteriologists; four members of the American Gynecological Society: Drs. Howard C. Taylor, Thomas Cullen, William E. Studdiford, Frank F. Simpson; four members of the American Surgical Association: Drs. George Brewer, Joseph Bloodgood, C. L. Gibson, Clement Cleveland; and Dr. S. Pollitzer of the American Dermatological Society. The laymen were Messrs. John E. Parsons, George C. Clark, James Speyer, V. Everit Macy, and Thomas M. Debevoise. Messrs. Clark and Debevoise were elected president and secretary. The mix of physicians and other health professionals with laymen has characterized the Society's boards of directors ever since, and has for many years been established in the bylaws as fifty-fifty.

page *15* Byzantine surgeons: M. B. Shimkin, *Contrary to Nature*. DHEW Publication no. (NIH)79-720 (Washington, D.C.: U.S. Government Printing Office, 1977), pp. 33–34.

page *16* "if we had seen the cases . . .": H. C. Taylor, "Educational Work in Carcinoma of the Uterus," *Transactions of the American Gynecological Society*, 1913, vol. 38, p. 453.

page *16* "In view of how little can be accomplished . . .": *Transactions of the American Gynecological Society*, 1903, vol. 28, p. 7.

page *16* "We used to hold consultations. . . .": *Cancer Control*. Report of an international symposium held at Lake Mohonk, N.Y., under the auspices of the ASCC (Chicago: Surgical Publishing Co., 1927), p. 164.

page *17* "You cannot get a number of physicians. . . .": F. L. Hoffman, "The Menace of Cancer," *Transactions of the American Gynecological Society*, 1913, vol. 38, p. 49.

page *17* ASCC's founders avoided professional education: D. F. Shaughnessy, "A History of the American Cancer Society." Ph.D. diss., Columbia University, 1955, p. 24. On file at American Cancer Society library, 4 West 35th Street, New York, N.Y. 10016.

page *18* "In 1905 when Dr. Lewis McMurtry . . .": *History of the American Society for the Control of Cancer, 1913–1943* (New York: New York City Cancer Committee, 1944), unpaginated.

page *19* "that this movement deserves the cooperation . . .": ASCC Minutes of the Executive Committee, (1913) I, p. 18.

page *20* "Dr. F. C. Wood reported that . . .": Shaughnessy, op. cit., p. 26.

page *20* "In places where the Society has been most active": Ibid.

page *20* "this condition can only be improved by . . .": Ibid., p. 25.

page *20* Elsie Mead and other lay founders: Ibid., p. 19.

page *21* "more than anyone else is responsible for . . .": Ibid., pp. 32–36.

page *21* "efforts should be first directed to . . .": Ibid., p. 29.

page *22* "The institution of a multiplicity of . . .": Ibid.

CHAPTER IV
Moving Up

page 23 Dr. Charles A. Powers set three axioms: D. F. Shaughnessy, *A History of the American Cancer Society*, op. cit., p. 39.

page 23 Danger Signals that May Mean Cancer: *History of the American Society for the Control of Cancer, 1913–1943*, op.cit., pp. dated 1921.

page 24 Mrs. Mead and membership drive: Shaughnessy, op. cit., pp. 36–42.

page 24 Journal of the American Medical Association editorial: Ibid., p. 56.

page 25 "It would be difficult to substantiate. . . .": Ibid., p. 94.

page 25 "spasmodic efforts to rouse the public.": Ibid.

page 25 Dr. Soper's outline of "Principles and Policies": Ibid., p. 96.

page 25 "There must be some middle ground between . . .": Ibid., p. 99.

page 26 "There must be no superficial examinations. . . .": Ibid., p. 55.

page 26 "with or without the cooperation of the local medical profession . . .": Ibid., p. 115.

page 27 "People are applying more promptly than . . .": Ibid., p. 79.

page 27 1927 survey by Dr. Raymond Brokaw: Ibid., p. 125–27.

CHAPTER V
Pullback and Advance

page 28 "a superficial program of lay publicity . . .": D. F. Shaughnessy, *A History of the American Cancer Society*, op. cit., pp. 139- 40.

page 29 "Existing facilities are entirely adequate. . . .": Ibid., pp. 141–42.

page 30 "The profession is inclined to view . . .": Ibid., p. 157.

page 31 "When the dead and dying from cancer . . .": Ibid., p. 176.

page 31 "In 1935 there were fifteen thousand . . .": Ibid., p. 142.

page 31 "inroads . . . on the prejudices . . .": Ibid., p. 134.

page 32 "to organize and administer the WFA . . .": Ibid., p. 183.

CHAPTER VI
Transformation

page 34 "A board of thirty is too large for . . .": D. F. Shaughnessy, *A History of the American Cancer Society*, op. cit., p. 149.

page 34 "There is an increasing pressure. . . .": Ibid., p. 151.

page 34 "The conquest of cancer will not be complete. . . .": Ibid., p. 206.

page 35 "infuriated when I read that there was . . .": Ibid., pp. 204–205.

page 35 "scattered over the nation and deeply concerned . . .": Ibid., p. 207.

page 36 "I got this money from Mr. Loewy. . . .": Ibid., pp. 215–16.

page 37 "As an advertising man . . .": E. Foote. Interview by author, Oct. 30, 1984. On file at American Cancer Society, Inc., 90 Park Avenue, New York, N.Y. 10016.

page *37* "Roughly, one out of six of you . . .": Ibid.

page *40* "it has made a breach in the wall of fear. . . .": Shaughnessy, op. cit., p. 192.

CHAPTER VII
The New Executive Vice-President

page *41* "Darned if I know. I was a banker . . .": L. W. Adams. Interview by author, Nov. 28, 1984. On file at American Cancer Society, Inc., 90 Park Avenue, New York, N.Y. 10016.

page *42* "Without my advice or consent or knowledge . . .": Ibid.

page *43* "I thought the job would only take about three years. . . .": Ibid.

page *43* "I was very disillusioned with what I found . . .": Ibid.

page *43* "It was not a very strong management team. . . .": Ibid.

CHAPTER VIII
The Smoking Gun

page *47* Death rates of smokers and nonsmokers: R. Pearl, "Tobacco Smoking and Longevity," *Science*, Mar. 4, 1938, vol. 87, p. 216.

page *47* "extensive scientific studies have proved that smoking . . .": Quoted in *The Dangers of Smoking; The Benefits of Quitting* (New York: American Cancer Society, Inc., 1972), p. 8.

page *47* A retrospective study is one that usually groups a number of patients with the same disease, and then attempts to find the probable cause by retracing their lives with regard to personal habits, the areas they lived in, their working conditions, and other environmental influences.

page *47* Studies done by M. Bouisson and F. E. Tylecote: H. S. Diehl, *Tobacco and Your Health* (New York: McGraw-Hill, 1969), pp. 16–17.

page *48* "Seventeen years elapsed. . . .": L. Breslow, *A History of Cancer Control in the United States. Book One.* DHEW Publication no. (NIH)79-1517 (Washington, D.C.: U.S. Government Printing Office, 1979), pp. 169–70.

page *49* "It's our conviction that the increase in the incidence . . .": Diehl, op. cit., p. 17.

page *49* "Extensive and prolonged use of tobacco . . .": E. L. Wynder and E. A. Graham, "Tobacco Smoking as a Possible Etiologic Factor in Bronchogenic Carcinoma," *Journal of the American Medical Association*, 1950, vol. 143, pp. 229–36.

page *50* "rising at an alarming rate . . .": E. C. Hammond. Interview by author, Oct. 22, 1984. On file at American Cancer Society, Inc., 90 Park Avenue, New York, N.Y. 10016.

page *52* "In 1950, when Hammond and Horn's study was . . .": R. Doll, "Smoking and Death Rates," *Journal of the American Medical Association*, 1984, vol. 251, p. 2854.

page 52 "an ability to collect unbiased information . . .": Ibid., p. 2855.

page 54 "Hammond and Horn's study broke new ground. . . .": Ibid., p. 2854.

CHAPTER IX

The Gun Goes Off

page 56 Hammond-Horn study: E. C. Hammond and D. Horn (with the assistance of L. Garfinkel, C. L. Percy, and L. Craig), "The Relationship Between Human Smoking Habits and Death Rates," *Journal of the American Medical Association*, 1954, vol. 155, pp. 1316–28.

page 56 "When it finally discovered that smoking was . . .": R. Carter, *The Gentle Legions* (Garden City, N.Y.: Doubleday, 1961), p. 163.

page 57 "available evidence indicates an association . . .": Quoted in Breslow, *A History of Cancer Control in the United States*, op. cit., p. 846.

page 58 "division within the board, whether we should be . . .": Adams. Interview, op. cit.

page 58 "We had a battle on the board of directors. . . .": Quoted in Breslow, op. cit., p. 849.

page 58 Hammond's study and Cameron's reaction: E. C. Hammond. Interview, op. cit.

page 58 "these lives are on my conscience. . . ." Breslow, op. cit., p. 846.

page 60 Dr. Leroy Burney's article: "The Weight of Evidence . . . Implicates Smoking as the Principal Etiological Factor in the Increasing Incidence of Lung Cancer," *Journal of the American Medical Association*, 1959, vol. 171, pp. 1829–37.

page 60 Cancer Prevention Study: *Cancer News* (Published by the American Cancer Society, Inc.), Fall 1971, vol. 25, pp. 17–19.

page 62 Study based on matched-pair analysis: E. C. Hammond, "Smoking in Relation to Mortality and Morbidity," *Journal of the National Cancer Institute*, 1964, vol. 32, pp. 1161–87.

CHAPTER X

The Government Joins the Battle

page 64 "The voluntary agencies have acted and used . . .": Letter to President John F. Kennedy, June 1, 1961. On file at American Cancer Society, Inc., 90 Park Avenue, New York, N.Y. 10016.

page 67 "Cigarette smoking is the major single cause . . .": *Report of the Surgeon General: The Health Consequences of Smoking, 1982*. (Washington, D.C.: U.S. Government Printing Office, 1982).

page 67 "cigarette smoking is a major cause of coronary heart disease. . . .": *Report of the Surgeon General: The Health Consequences of Smoking, 1983*. (Washington, D.C.: U.S. Government Printing Office, 1983), pp. 6–7.

page 71 Smoking-dogs experiments: E. C. Hammond, O. Auerbach, D.

Kirman, and L. Garfinkel, "Effects of Cigarette Smoking on Dogs," *Archives of Environmental Health*, Dec. 1970, vol. 21, p. 752.

page 75 Weighted sales average is the amount of tar and nicotine in each brand in proportion to total sales.

page 75 "The Society [ACS] must be credited with . . .": Carter, *The Gentle Legions, op. cit., p. 164.*

CHAPTER XI
The Cell Yields a Secret

page 76 "no specific symptoms [to rely upon] for early diagnosis . . .": Breslow, *A History of Cancer Control in the United States*, op. cit., p. 197. Based on a paper delivered by Dr. Ewing to the First International Symposium on Cancer, held by the ASCC in 1926.

page 78 "The experiments required obtaining the ova of the female guinea pigs. . . .": D. E. Carmichael, *The Pap Smear* (Springfield, Ill.: Charles C. Thomas, 1973), pp. 47–48.

page 78 "The females of all higher animals have a . . .": Ibid., p. 48.

page 79 "an impressive wealth of diverse cell forms . . .": Ibid.

page 80 "The Diagnosis of Early Human Pregnancy . . .": *Proceedings of the Society for Experimental Biology and Medicine*, 1925, vol. 22, pp. 436–37.

page 80 "It was inevitable that among these . . .": Carmichael, op. cit., p. 56.

page 80 "failed to convince my colleagues of the . . .": Ibid., p. 61.

page 81 "Dr. Papanicolaou expressed his previous discouragement. . . .": Ibid., p. 68.

page 81 "by use of the vaginal smear . . .": Ibid., p. 69.

page 81 "if this proves diagnostic in a large number of cases . . .": Ibid., pp. 69–70.

CHAPTER XII
The Selling of the Cell

page 84 "I was on the [surgical] staff of Memorial. . . .": C. S. Cameron. Interview by author, Dec. 31, 1984. On file at American Cancer Society, Inc., 90 Park Avenue, New York, N.Y. 10016.

page 84 "[As] a result of my conversations with Dr. Papanicolaou . . ." Breslow, *A History of Cancer Control in the United States*, op. cit., p. 221.

page 85 "I think that perhaps did something to persuade . . .": Ibid.

page 86 "The Pap Smear isn't diagnosing cancer. . . .": Ibid., p. 227.

page 86 "I was young and single. . . .": A. I. Holleb. Interview by author, Sept. 13, 1984. On file at American Cancer Society, Inc.

page 87 "There were many people in the Cancer Society medical group. . . .": Cameron Interview, op. cit.

page *88* "in view of the poorly understood changes . . . .": Minutes of the American Cancer Society Medical and Scientific Committee, June 15, 1951.

page *88* "We need not wait for more evidence. . . . .": Minutes of the American Cancer Society Annual Meeting, Nov. 1951.

page *88* The ACS currently recommends that women at normal risk be given the Pap test annually for two years. If both tests are negative, the test should be repeated every two or three years thereafter. However, the physician must make the determination in each individual case as to how often the test is needed.

page *89* "Dr. Papanicolaou credited Dr. Cameron. . . . .": Carmichael, op. cit., p. 76.

page *89* "The thing was timed pretty well. . . . .": Cameron interview, op. cit.

page *89* "You were supposed to tell your doctor. . . . .": Holleb Interview, op. cit.

page *90* "Cytology was not the only factor in reducing . . .": Cameron Interview, op. cit.

page *90* "faster and probably better than the mass application . . .": L. Koss. Interview, 1976. Quoted in Breslow, op. cit., p. 243.

page *91* "whether Papanicolaou smears are effective in reducing . . .": B. Stenkvist, R. Bergstrom, G. Eklund, and C. H. Fox, "Papanicolaou Smear Screening and Cervical Cancer," *Journal of the American Medical Association*, 1984, vol. 252, pp. 1423–26.

page *92* Survival rates for uterine cancer: *1985 Cancer Facts & Figures* (New York: American Cancer Society, Inc., 1985), p. 11.

page *92* Various uses of exfoliative cytology: Based on *Report of the National Panel of Consultants on the Conquest of Cancer*, op. cit., p. 42.

CHAPTER XIII

Breast Cancer: Can Women Be Protected?

page *94* Lung-cancer deaths are more numerous despite the fact that incidence is much lower than that of breast cancer. The reason: The overall five-year survival rate of lung cancer patients is only 12 percent, as against 72-percent survival for breast-cancer patients. The explanation: Lung cancer, unlike breast cancer, is extremely difficult to detect early, and to cure.

page *95* "there is increasing clinical, pathologic, and epidemiologic . . .": G. P. Murphy, ed., *Cancer Signals and Safeguards* (Littleton, Mass.: PSG Publishing, 1980), p. 119.

page *95* "Physicians engaged in the practice of oncology . . .": A. I. Holleb, "The Purposes and Goals of Breast Self-Examination," *Cancer Bulletin*, 1979, vol. 31, no. 5, p. 136.

page *96* "We were seeing altogether too many cases. . . . .": A. M. Popma. Interview by author, Apr. 4, 1985, and typewritten narrative dated 1952. Both on file at American Cancer Society, Inc., 90 Park Avenue, New York, N.Y. 10016.

page 99 "There are no great disagreements about skin dosage. . . .": Breslow, *A History of Cancer Control in the United States*, op. cit., p. 293.

CHAPTER XIV
Breast X-Ray: Can it Save Lives?

page 101 "most effective program for earlier detection then available . . ." Holleb Interview, op. cit.

page 101 "The American Cancer Society deems it part of our steward-ship. . . .": A. I. Holleb. Letter to U.S. Congressman Henry A. Waxman, Calif., May 31, 1977. On file at American Cancer Society, Inc., 90 Park Avenue, New York, N.Y. 10016.

page 102 "totally disinterested and wanted no part. . . .": Breslow, op. cit., p. 297.

page 104 "Unexpectedly, the widespread use of mammography . . .": L. W. Bassett and R. H. Gold, in *Mammography, Thermography and Ultrasound in Breast Cancer Detection* (New York: Grune & Stratton, 1982), p. 4.

page 104 "I regretfully conclude that there seems to be . . .": B. C. Bailar, "Mammography: A Contrary View," *Annals of Internal Medicine*, 1976, vol. 84, pp. 77–84.

page 105 "the [BCDDP] program contains seeds of a major disaster. . . .": D. S. Greenberg and J. E. Randal, "Waging the Wrong War Against Cancer," *Washington Post*, May 1, 1977.

page 106 "[While] recent epidemiologic studies suggest . . .": National Cancer Institute, Background statement on X-ray mammography, July 19, 1976.

page 106 "These were women who needed mammograms. . . .": A. I. Holleb. Interview on CBS Television Network, Aug. 27, 1976. Transcript distributed by American Cancer Society, Inc., Sept. 3, 1976.

page 107 "To physicians, these figures meant that . . .": W. S. Ross, "What Every Woman Should Know About Breast X-Ray," *Reader's Digest*, Mar. 1977. Based on a 1976 interview with Dr. Benjamin F. Byrd, Jr., president of the American Cancer Society, Inc.

page 107 "Between thirty-five and fifty, the vast majority of women . . .": Holleb. TV Interview, op. cit.

CHAPTER XV
"Purposeless Mutilations"?

page 108 "ascertain what scientific information could be obtained . . .": Operational Memorandum no. 6, Breast Cancer Detection Demonstration Project, May 3, 1977.

page 108 "The Cancer Society is expected to acquiesce. . . .": "Mammography Muddle," Editorial, *New York Times*, May 12, 1977.

page 109 "More than 2,109 unsuspected breast cancers . . .": A. I. Holleb, Letter to the *New York Times*, June 2, 1977.

page 109 I. D. J. Bross and N. Natarajan, "Genetic Damage from Diagnostic Radiation," *Journal of the American Medical Association*, 1977, Vol. 237, pp. 2390–2401.

page 109 "This exposure [in BCDDP] to diagnostic X-ray . . .": D. S. Greenberg and J. E. Randal, "Waging the Wrong War Against Cancer," op. cit.

page 110 "false and unsubstantiated . . .": Statement of the American Cancer Society, Inc. (undated), issued with Interorganization Memorandum DE-85, Feb. 17, 1978.

page 110 "women had their breasts wholly or partly removed. . . .": "Mammography Mistake," Editorial, *New York Times*, Sept. 25, 1977.

page 110 "pathology is not part of the screening projects. . . .": A. I. Holleb, "Mammography Is Not a Mistake," Letter to *New York Times*, Oct. 8, 1977.

page 111 "The mammography war isn't over. . . .": "Ultra-low Mammography Doses Challenge Latest Guidelines," *Medical World News*, Nov. 14, 1977, p. 14.

page 111 "purposeless mutilation had been inflicted. . . .": D. S. Greenberg, "Perils in a Cancer Screening Project," *Washington Post*, Oct. 10, 1978.

page 112 "traces back to the American Cancer Society . . .": Ibid.

page 112 "the hospitals had preferred to keep their original slides. . . .": "Those 'Needless' Mastectomies: Were there 66, or Fewer, or None?" *Medical World News*, Nov. 28, 1977, pp. 7–8.

page 113 "great care was given to the diagnosis and management. . . .": O. H. Beahrs, S. Shapiro, and C. Smart, *Supplemental and Concluding Report of the Working Group to Review the NCI/ACS Breast Cancer Detection Demonstration Projects*. NCI Contract RFP-N01-CN-75379, Aug. 18, 1978, p. 12.

CHAPTER XVI
Developing a Clearer Picture

page 114 "reduced-dose film mammography (or xeroradiography) . . .": O. H. Beahrs, S. Shapiro, and C. Smart, *Supplemental and Concluding Report*, op. cit., p. 21.

page 114 "remarkable that, regardless of age . . .": L. H. Baker, *Breast Cancer Detection Demonstration Project: Five Year Summary Report (New York: American Cancer Society, Inc., 1982), p. 6.*

page 114 "Women over 50 should have a mammogram. . . .": "New ACS Guidelines for Cancer Checkups," *Cancer News* (American Cancer Society, Inc.), Spring/Summer 1980, vol. 34, p. 22.

page 114 "Of the 4,443 cancers recorded in the BCDDP . . .": Baker, op. cit., p. 35.

page 116 "The criticism of mammography as a diagnostic . . .": G. D. Dodd, "Mammography, State of the Art," in *Proceedings: National Conference on Breast Cancer* (New York: American Cancer Society, 1983), p. 652.

page 116 "The serious import of breast cancer lies in . . .": P. Strax, "Mass Screening for Control of Breast Cancer," ibid., pp. 665–70.

page 116 Cancer-Related Checkup Guidelines for mammography: *Mammography Guidelines 1983: Background Statement and Update of Cancer-Related Checkup Guidelines for Breast Cancer Detection in Asymptomatic Women Age 40 to 49.* Reprinted from *CA: A Cancer Journal for Clinicians* (New York: American Cancer Society, 1983).

page 117 AMA recommendations for mammography: *Journal of the American Medical Association,* 1984, vol. 252, pp. 3008–11.

CHAPTER XVII

Cancer Research: The Black Hole

page 122 "I am absolutely convinced that the cancer death rate . . .": M. R. Runyon, "The American Cancer Society: A Profile." Address given at the Biltmore Hotel, New York, N.Y., Oct. 25, 1959 (New York: American Cancer Society, Inc., 1959), p. 4. (See Appendix A.)

page 122 "Our Society was founded for lay education. . . .": H. C. Taylor, "Thirty Years of Cancer Control," *Quarterly Review,* Oct. 1943, vol. 8, p. 39.

page 122 "conduct researches, investigations, experiments . . ." Senate Bill 2067, 75th Congress, in Breslow, op. cit.

page 123 The Committee on Growth began its attack: *American Cancer Society Research Report* (New York: American Cancer Society, 1984), p. 1.

CHAPTER XVIII

Research: The End of Cancer

page 125 "After centuries of bewilderment . . .": J. M. Bishop, Acceptance Remarks, 1982 (37th Annual) Albert Lasker Medical Research Awards Luncheon, New York, N.Y.

page 126 Quotes of optimism among cancer experts: From P. Boffey, "No More Cancer by the Year 2128?" *New York Times,* Feb. 20, 1983. Reprinted in *Cancer News,* Spring/Summer 1983, vol. 37, pp. 12–13.

page 128 "In cells DNA is transcribed into a strand. . . .": J. M. Bishop, "Oncogenes," *Scientific American,* Mar. 1982, vol. 246, pp. 80–92.

page 129 "This suggests that the design of rational therapeutic . . .": Ibid.

page 130 "To answer that question, Milstein and Kohler . . .": J. L. Fox, "Antibody Reagents Revolutionizing Immunology," *Chemical & Engineering News,* Jan. 1, 1975, p. 15.

page 131 "A sixty-seven-year-old man at Stanford . . .": R. A. Miller, D. G. Maloney, R. Warnke, and R. Levy, "Treatment of B-Cell Lymphoma with Monoclonal Anti-Odiotype Antibodies," *New England Journal of Medicine,* 1982, vol. 306, pp. 517–522.

page 132 "We try to use our research funds not merely as . . .": F. R. Rauscher.

Interview by author, Nov. 19, 1984. On file at American Cancer Society, Inc., 90 Park Avenue, New York, N.Y., 10016

CHAPTER XIX

Clinical Research: To Help the Cancer Patient

page 143 "there is evidence that the pace quickens. . . .": C. G. Zubrod, "Development of Anti-Cancer Therapy," in J. H. Burchenal and H. F. Oettgen, eds., *Cancer Achievements, Challenges and Prospects for the 1980's*, vol. 2 (New York: Grune & Stratton, 1981), p. 1.

page 143 "Clinical investigation is essentially the culmination of . . .": *Report of the National Panel of Consultants on the Conquest of Cancer*, op. cit., p. 23.

page 144 "to close the gap between what we know and . . .": Quoted in Breslow, *A History of Cancer Control in the United States*, op. cit., p. 1.

page 144 "I have a right to expect and I think . . .": Ibid., pp. 14–15.

page 144 "Cancer patients—and the doctors treating them . . .": V. T. DeVita, *The Cancer Letter*, Oct. 23, 1981, vol. 7, pp. 3–4.

page 145 "However, even when the surgeon and the radiation oncologist . . .": Zubrod, "Development of Anti-Cancer Therapy," op. cit., pp. 2–3.

page 146 "Drugs that could cause remission . . ."' Ibid. p. 3.

page 146 "Surgery and radiotherapy are limited not only by . . .": Quoted in Breslow, op. cit., p. 408. Cure of Hodgkin's disease: E. C. Easson, "The Cure of Hodgkin's Disease," *British Medical Journal*, 1963, vol. 1, pp. 1704–07.

page 151 "The understanding and management of patients with . . .": S. A. Rosenberg, "Advances in the Treatment of Malignant Lymphomas," in Burchenal and Oettinger, eds., *Cancer Achievements, Challenges and Prospects*, op. cit., p. 419.

CHAPTER XX

ACS International

page 153 Worldwide frequency of cancers 1975: D. M. Parkin, J. Stjernsward, and C. S. Muir, "Estimates of the Worldwide Frequency of Twelve Major Cancers," *Bulletin of the World Health Organization*, 1984, vol. 62, no. 2, pp. 163–82.

page 155 "the investigation of what other countries were doing . . .": Shaughnessy, *A History of the American Cancer Society*, op. cit., p. 83.

page 155 "practical fact or sound working opinions . . .": Ibid., p. 87.

page 155 International cancer research and control (UICC): M. E. Allen, *Historical Perspectives of the Committee to Advance the Worldwide Fight Against Cancer*. Pamphlet (New York: American Cancer Society, Nov. 18, 1977), p. 3.

page 156 "We have to do something to help other . . .": Ibid., p. 4.
page 156 "to aid and stimulate the creation of cancer societies . . .": Ibid.
page 156 "It is fair to say that in my three years . . .": Ibid., p. 10.

CHAPTER XXI

Reach to Recovery

page 161 "In 1952, during my most frightening . . .": T. Lasser, *Reach to Recovery* (New York: American Cancer Society, 1974), p. 6.
page 162 "Pain lances through the numbness that is your body. . . .": T. Lasser and W. K. Clarke, *Reach to Recovery* (New York: Simon & Schuster, 1972), p. 18.
page 163 "In our bosom-oriented culture . . .": A. I. Holleb, Foreword to Lasser and Clarke, *Reach to Recovery*, Ibid., p. 9.
page 164 "When I walked into the hospital room . . .": Lasser, *Reach to Recovery* (American Cancer Society), op. cit., pp. 7–8.
page 164 "I'm running late, I've been on the go. . . .": Ibid., p. 8.
page 164 " 'You haven't gone through what I have' . . .": Ibid.
page 164 "At that precise moment, I think . . .": Ibid.
page 167 "Many surgeons looked upon the program as . . .": A. I. Holleb, "The Reach to Recovery Program of the American Cancer Society," report at Sixteenth Annual International GBK Symposium, Düsseldorf, West Germany, July 5–7, 1984.
page 170 French attitude toward breast amputation: Fi Timothy. Interview by author, Feb. 13, 1985. On file at American Cancer Society, Inc., 90 Park Avenue, New York, N.Y. 10016.
page 170 "And she was so grateful when I left . . .": F. Timothy, Interview by author, ibid.
page 171 "In the beginning, at least eighty percent . . .": Ibid.

CHAPTER XXII

The Warm Hand of Service to Patients: Volunteers Create Their Own Programs

page 174 "One of our jobs is to find people. . . .": Quoted in J. C. Snidecor et al., *Speech Rehabilitation of the Laryngectomized* (Springfield, Ill.: Charles C. Thomas, 1969), p. 11.
page 174 "In the mid 1970s, I was beginning to see . . .": J. Johnson. Interview by author, Apr. 26, 1985.
page 177 CanSurmount chapters: "CanSurmount: Patients Helping Patients," *Cancer News*, Spring 1978, vol. 32, pp. 11–12; and D. Fink, "The ACS and Human Concerns," *Cancer News*, Winter 1983, vol. 37, pp. 8–11.

CHAPTER XXIII
Life After Cancer

page 180   "There's a new excitement in the ranks of . . .": L. W. Adams, Opening Remarks, in *Proceedings: National Conference on Human Values and Cancer* (New York: American Cancer Society, 1973), p. 12.

page 181   "Are patients any the worse physically for their . . .": B. C. Byrd, Jr., "The People Side of Cancer," in *Proceedings: National Conference on Human Values and Cancer*, ibid., pp. 16–17.

page 181   "A Conference such as this places in proper perspective . . .": A. I. Holleb, "Conference Summation and the Future," in *Proceedings: National Conference on Human Values and Cancer*, ibid., p. 181.

page 182   "All of us want to live with dignity. . . .": A. I. Holleb, "You Are Not Alone—You Are Not Alone," Report on Second Conference on Human Values and Cancer, *Cancer News*, Winter 1978, vol. 32, pp. 4–5.

CHAPTER XXIV
Affirmative Action: Cancer in Minorities

page 184   "We devised a committee on community involvement. . . .": L. D. Leffall, Jr. Interview by author, Nov. 7, 1985. On file at American Cancer Society, Inc.

page 184   "It was the right time, the 1960's. . . .": Ibid.

page 186   "there is some connection between the low economic . . .": Quoted by J. H. Jones, Press Release (undated), ACS Fourteenth Science Writers' Seminar, Mar. 24–29, 1972.

page 186   "All of us are aware of the difficulties in . . .": J. H. Jones and A. J. Dixon, Memorandum to Mr. Lane W. Adams, "Involvement of Minorities in the ACS," July 6, 1977.

page 188   "We must meet the challenge of cancer among black . . .": L. D. Leffall, Jr., Address given at the Conference on Challenge of Cancer Among Black Americans, Feb. 17, 1979.

page 189   "The black population is comprised of a . . .": H. P. Freeman, "Affirmative Action to Save Black Lives," *Cancer News*, Spring/Summer 1981, vol. 35, pp. 7, 18.

page 189   "The most dramatic improvement in cancer mortality . . .": Ibid.

CHAPTER XXV
Crusade

page 196   " 'You've got cancer of the larynx,' he said. . . .": W. Gargan and A. Hano, *Why Me?* (Garden City, N.Y.: Doubleday, 1965).

CHAPTER XXVI

United Way or a Better Way?

page 198 "This created much dissension. . . .": F. E. Wilcox. Interview by author, Nov. 8, 1984. On file at American Cancer Society, Inc., 90 Park Avenue, New York, N.Y. 10016.

page 199 "those in the United Way were raising only half . . .": T. Ulmer. Interview by author, Nov. 8, 1984. On file at American Cancer Society, Inc.

page 200 "The United Way wanted to retain them as . . .": Wilcox Interview, op. cit.

page 202 "When you were receiving money with little effort . . .": Adams Interview, op. cit.

page 203 "However, there was no way we could submit. . . .": Ibid.

page 203 "He knew if we were ever to have any . . .": Ibid.

page 203 "People in industry needed our educational programs. . . .": L. W. Adams, Remarks to ACS Eastern Area, Sept. 1979.

page 204 "Aramony's neck was way out on this. . . .": Adams Interview, op. cit.

page 204 "I told Mr. Jonas who it was. . . .": Ibid.

page 205 Authority to make new agreements with United Way: Minutes of the American Cancer Society Board of Directors, Nov. 8, 1980.

CHAPTER XXVII

". . . Without Representation"

page 206 "It was like the early days in the United States. . . .": Wilcox Interview, op. cit.

page 206 "This led to some of the divisions not having any . . .": T. Carlile, *The American Cancer Society: Oct. 1961–Oct. 1962*. Memoir prepared at request of R. Lee Clark, former president of American Cancer Society, as part of current history of ACS presidents, 1983. On file at American Cancer Society, Inc., 90 Park Avenue, New York, N.Y. 10016.

page 206 "As the Society grew, there was a perception. . . .": Wilcox Interview, op. cit.

page 207 "In 1959, President Warren Cole first appointed . . .": Carlile, op. cit.

page 207 "discussion was hot and heavy. . . .": C. R. Ebersol. Interview by author, Nov. 4, 1984. On file at American Cancer Society, Inc.

page 208 "After discussion (which required seven pages of minutes) . . ."; Carlile, op. cit.

page 208 "It was lay leadership that carried on the fight. . . .": Wilcox Interview, op. cit.

page 208 "Dr. Pendergrass chaired the committee again. . . .": Carlile, op. cit.

page 208 "It brought a greater representation of divisions. . . .": R. P. McGrail. Interview by author, Jan. 2, 1985. On file at American Cancer Society, Inc.

page 209 "They all report to the board. . . .": Adams Interview, op. cit.

page 209 "We almost split apart on the issue of structure. . . .": Wilcox Interview, op. cit.

CHAPTER XXVIII

Cancer Becomes a National Priority: The National Cancer Acts

page 210 "When I asked my husband for money for the American Cancer Society . . .": Lasker Interview, op. cit.

page 211 "The danger of putting the government in a dominant . . .": Quoted in Breslow, *A History of Cancer Control in the United States*, op. cit., p. 510.

page 213 "The Lasker fortune could have established a research . . .": M. B. Shimkin, *As Memory Serves: Six Essays on a Personal Involvement with the National Cancer Institute, 1938 to 1978.* NIH Publication no. 83–2217 (Washington, D.C.: U.S. Government Printing Office, 1983), p. 38.

page 213 "Mary Lasker occupies and will be remembered for . . .": Ibid.

page 214 NCI budget increase: *Fact Sheet, National Cancer Institute, Mar. 1985.* (Washington, D.C.: U.S. Government Printing Office, 1985), p. 21.

page 214 "It would take one billion dollars a year. . . .": Quoted in Breslow, op. cit., p. 705, based on an interview with former senator Yarborough by Devra Breslow in 1977.

page 215 "supported by fifty-three of my colleagues in the Senate . . .": Foreword, *Report of the National Panel of Consultants on the Conquest of Cancer*, op. cit., p. xiii.

page 216 "The committee is unanimously of the view that . . .": Ibid., p. xv.

page 216 "the unanimous sense of the Congress . . .": Quoted in Breslow, op. cit., p. 708.

page 217 "Failure of cellular mechanisms to eradicate . . .": *Report of the National Panel of Consultants on the Conquest of Cancer*, op. cit., p. 25.

page 218 "may enjoy a pharmacological sanctuary where . . .": Ibid., p. 26.

page 219 The Conquest of Cancer bill: R. A. Rettig, *Cancer Crusade* (Princeton, N.J.: Princeton University Press, 1977), p. 121.

page 220 "it would be a wonderful idea. . . .": Ibid., p. 122.

page 220 "the necessary administrative setup would not be easy. . . .": *Report of the National Panel of Consultants on the Conquest of Cancer*, op. cit., p. 4.

CHAPTER XXIX

Public Issues

page 224 "areas of dialogue regarding the interface . . .": A. C. Davis. Interview by author, Oct. 23, 1984. Transcript and tapes on file at American Cancer Society, Inc., 90 Park Avenue, New York, N.Y. 10016.

page 226 "The Toxic Substances Control Act of 1976 . . .": A. C. Davis. Personal Memorandum to W. S. Ross, Oct. 31, 1985. On file at American Cancer Society, Inc.

page 226 "there was some concern that President Ford might veto . . .": ACS Memorandum, and B. F. Byrd, Jr., Letter, Sept. 29, 1976.

page 228 "places the emphasis on diagnosis and cures . . .": Greenberg and Randal, "Waging the Wrong War Against Cancer," op. cit.

page 228 "As an organization started and directed by volunteers . . .": R. L. Clark, and F. J. Rauscher, "Cancer: A Search for Both Cures and Causes," *Washington Post*, May 12, 1977.

page 229 Hearings held under Chairman L. H. Fountain: U.S. Congress, House, Subcommittee of the Committee on Government Operations, *Hearings on the National Cancer Institute, 95th Congress, 2nd sess. June 1977*. 94-577 0 (Washington, D.C.: U.S. Government Printing Office, 1977), p. 2.

page 229 "Are we spending our money as effectively as . . .": J. W. Wydler, ibid., p. 4.

page 230 "The relationship is close, but . . .": Davis, Memorandum, op. cit.

page 232 "We have no evidence that saccharin causes cancer. . . .": R. D. Lyons, "Proposed Saccharin Ban Backed by the F.D.A. at Hearing in House," *New York Times*, Mar. 22, 1977.

page 233 "level of tolerable risk": J. Fritsch, "Ex-FDA commissioner urges law to OK saccharin," *Chicago Tribune*, May 11, 1977.

page 233 "as a major national voluntary health agency . . .": American Cancer Society statement on saccharin, Nov. 1980.

page 234 Composition of Public Issues Committee: Article VI, Committees of the Board of Directors, Bylaws of the American Cancer Society, Nov. 1977, amended.

CHAPTER XXX

The Record

page 236 "the control and eradication of cancer": *American Cancer Society: What It Is; What It Does; How It Began; Where It Is Going*. (New York, American Cancer Society, 1977), p. 2.

Indexes

Index of Names

A

Adair, Frank, 36, 38, 161, 163, 164, 165
Adams, Elaine, 42, 43
Adams, James, 36, 38, 42, 51, 58
Adams, Lane W., 41, 42, 43, 58, 59,
    134, 167, 179, 180, 182, 183, 186,
    187, 188, 195, 197, 198, 201, 203,
    204, 209, 224, 234
Adams, Samuel Hopkins, 19
Aetios of Amida, 15
Allen, Mildred E., 155, 156
Amida, Aetios of, *see* Aetios of Amida
Anderson, Karen, xv
Aramony, William, 203, 204
Arthur D. Little & Co., 234
Atwater, W. O., 245
Auerbach, Oscar, 70
Avery, Arch, 196, 197

B

Bahnzaf, John, 70
Bailar, John C. III, 102, 103, 104, 105,
    106, 111, 227
Baker, Carl, 224
Baker, Larry H., 114
Baltimore, David, 233, 234
Bayh, Marvella, 196
Bayne-Jones, Stanhope, 65
Beahrs, Oliver, 108, 110, 111, 112, 113,
    114
Beggan, Robert, 203
Bentsen, Lloyd, 219
Berlin, Nathaniel, 103
Bernstein, Carl, 227
Billroth, Christian Albert Theodor, 16
Bishop, J. Michael, 125, 126, 127, 128,
    129

Black, Herbert, 181
Blake, Amanda, 195, 196
Bland-Sutton, John, 16
Blatnick, Jeff, 194
Bobst, Elmer, 36, 38, 42, 51, 58, 155,
    156, 157, 219, 220
Bone, Hugh, 211
Bouisson, M., 47
Brainard, Morgan, 36
Brandt, Edward N., Jr., 67
Braniff, Thomas, 36
Breslow, Lester, 107
Brokaw, Raymond, 27
Bross, Irwin, 109, 110, 227
Bryant, Joseph L., 242
Burchenal, Joseph H., 146
Burdette, Walter J., 65
Burney, Leroy, 60
Byrd, Benjamin F., Jr., 107, 180, 181,
    182, 226, 234, 235

C

Cameron, Charles S., 15, 50, 51, 58,
    77, 84, 85, 86, 87, 88, 89, 90
Cantell, K., 133, 134
Carbone, Paul P., 151
Cardwell, John J., 188
Carlile, Thomas, 99, 206, 207, 208
Carmichael, E., 78, 80, 81, 83
Carson, Rachel, 225
Carter, Richard, 56, 58, 75
Casey, Lee, 35, 36, 37
Childe, C. P., 18
Chittenden, R. H., 245
Clark, George C., 6, 21
Clark, John, 18
Clark, R(andolph) Lee, 157, 214, 215,
    228, 232, 235

Cleveland, Clement, 20, 242
Cline, John W., 64
Cochran, William G., 65
Coggeshall, Lowell, 200
Cohen, Jacob Gershon-, see Gershon-
    Cohen, Jacob
Cole, Warren, 99, 207
Comer, George W., 79
Comer, Jonathan, 188
Compton, Arthur H., 212
Conant, James B., 212
Cooper, Geoffrey, 128
Copeland, Murray, 99
Cornelia, Paul, 184
Crowell, Herman, 31
Cullen, Thomas S., 18, 19, 241
Cutler, Sidney J., 188

D

Davies, Lawrence E., 53
Davis, Alan, 102, 223, 224, 226, 230,
    234
Davis, Byron B., 26
DeBakey, Michael, 212
Debevoise, Thomas, 21, 25
Deep Throat, 227
de Harven, Gerry Schramm, 156
Denoix, Pierre, 155, 170
d'Estaing, Valery Giscard, see Giscard
    d'Estaing, Valery
de Tocqueville, Alexis, see Tocqueville,
    Alexis de
DeVita, Vincent T., 127, 144, 151
DeYoung, Herbert C., 64
Diebert, Austin, 97
Diehl, Harold S., 43
Dixon, Agnes J., 186
Dock, George, 48
Dodd, Gerald D., 116
Doll, Richard, 52, 54
Douglas, Kirk, 196
Douglas, Lewis, 36
Dunbar, Mrs. S. O., 32

E

Eason, Eric C., 148
Ebersol, Charles R., xv, 157, 207, 234,
    235
Edwards, Ralph, 196
Egan, Robert, 99

Eisenhower, Dwight D., xvi
Epstein, Samuel, 227
Erikson, Raymond L., 126
Erlichman, John, 220
Estaing, Valery Giscard d', see Giscard
    d'Estaing, Valery
Ewing, James, 25, 76, 212

F

Farber, Emmanuel, 65
Farber, Sidney, 213, 215
Farrand, Livingston, 17
Faulkner, William, xiv
Feiser, Louis F., 65
Fisher, Bernard, 147
Flood, David, 144
Fogarty, John E., 212, 214
Foote, Emerson, 35, 36, 37, 42, 212,
    215
Ford, Betty (Mrs. Gerald R.), xv, 104
Ford, Gerald R., 104, 226
Forsythe, John, 196
Fountain, L. H., 229
Fox, J. L., 130
Freeman, Harold P., 188, 189
Funston, G. Keith, 219
Furth, Jacob, 65

G

Gadberry, G. Robert, 195
Gallo, Robert C., 126, 136, 137
Garb, Solomon, 220
Gardner, Warren H., 173
Garfinkel, Lawrence, 52, 53, 60, 65, 70,
    185
Gargan, Bill, 196
Gershon-Cohen, Jacob, 98, 99
Gilbert, Rene, 148
Giscard d'Estaing, Valery, 171
Graham, Evarts A., 49
Graham, Otto, 195
Graham, Ruth, 84
Graham, Virginia, xv, 195
Graves, Peter, 196
Green, C. E., 245
Greenberg, Daniel S., 111, 112, 223,
    228, 229, 230
Gressor, Ian, 133
Gutterman, Jordan, 133, 134

H

Haagensen, C. D., 97
Haeckel, Ernst, 77
Hagman, Larry, xv
Hamilton, Paul K., 176, 177
Hammond, E. Cuyler, 47, 49, 50, 51,
    52, 53, 54, 55, 56, 57, 58, 60, 61,
    65, 66, 69, 70, 73, 90, 235
Hammond, Marian (Mrs. E. Cuyler), 51
Hanafusa, Hidesaburo, 125
Harris, W. J., 20
Heidelberger, Charles, 146
Hektoen, Ludvig, 212
Heller, John R., 144
Hickam, John H., 65
Higginson, John, 154, 230
Hill, Lister, 214, 215
Hinsey, Joseph, 81, 82
Hoffman, Anna Rosenberg, 212, 215
Hoffman, Frederick L., 18, 20, 121,
    122, 242, 244
Holleb, Arthur I., 77, 86, 89, 95, 101,
    102, 103, 106, 107, 109, 110, 163,
    167, 168, 179, 180, 181, 182, 184,
    186, 224, 232
Hope, Bob, 33
Horn, Daniel, 51, 52, 53, 54, 55, 56,
    57, 58, 66, 67, 69, 73
Horne, Lena, xv, 187
Horsch, Kathleen (Mrs. Lawrence J.),
    195
Horsley, Victor, 16
Humphrey, Hubert H., 156
Hutchinson, William B., 215

I

Illig, Marjorie G., 30, 40

J

Jackson, Dudley, 211
Janvrin, J. E., 16
Jason, Robert, 184
Javits, Jacob K., 219, 220, 221
Johnson, Judi, 174, 175, 176
Johnston, Eric, 36
Jonas, Allan K., 195, 204
Jones, John Henry, 185, 186

Jones, Stanhope Bayne-, see Bayne-
    Jones, Stanhope
Jones, Walter, 42
Jordan, Vernon E., Jr., 187

K

Kaplan, Henry S., 149, 150
Kaye, Danny, 196
Keith, Jeff, 194
Kennedy, Edward M., 215, 219, 220,
    221
Kennedy, John F., 64
Kissner, Janice, 188
Kohler, George, 130
Kohler, Walter, 42
Koss, Leopold, 90, 91
Krim, Mathilde, 215

L

Lamont, Thomas W., 21
Landers, Ann, 196, 220
Lasker, Albert D., 33, 35, 36, 37, 38,
    58, 193, 210, 212, 213
Lasker, Mary (Mrs. Albert D.), 33, 35,
    36, 37, 42, 122, 134, 156, 157, 193,
    210, 211, 212, 213, 215, 219, 220
Lasser, J. K., 166
Lasser, Terese, 161, 162, 163, 164, 165,
    166, 167, 168, 169, 172
Lawson, Mrs. R. C., 32
Leffall, LaSalle D., Jr., 183, 184, 185,
    186, 187, 188, 190
LeMaistre, Charles, 65
Letton, A. Hamblin, 180
Levy, Ronald, 131, 132
Lewis, William, 213
Little, Arthur D. & Co., see Arthur D.
    Little & Co.
Little, Clarence Cook, 28, 29, 30, 31,
    33, 34, 35, 38, 40, 211, 212
Littler, Gene, 195
Loewy, Raymond, 36
Logan, Wende W., 111

M

McDivitt, Robert W., 110, 111, 112
McGrail, Richard P., 203, 208
McKinsey & Co., 223, 225

McMurtry, Lewis, 18, 241
Macy, V. Everit, 21
Magnusson, Warren, 211
Markel, William, 167, 180
Mars, Audrey, 157
Maverick, Maury, 211
Mavroyeni, Mary, see Papanicolaou, Mary (Mrs. George N.)
Mayo, William J., 22
Mead, Elsie (Mrs. Robert G.), 20, 21, 24, 183, 242
Meigs, Joe, 84
Marigan, Thomas, 133, 134
Miller, Lois Mattox, 37
Milligan, Lucy, 40
Milstein, Cesar, 130
Morton, John J., Jr., 38
Murphy, Gerald P., 38, 157
Murayama, H., 82, 83, 89

N

Nelson, Gaylord, 221
Newell, Guy R., Jr., 230, 232
Nixon, Richard M., 194, 220, 221
Norby, Pat, 175

O

Ochsner, Alton, 48, 59

P

Papanicolaou, George N., 76, 77, 78, 79, 80, 81, 82, 83, 84, 85, 86, 87, 88, 89
Papanicolaou, Mary (Mrs. George N.), 77, 78, 79
Papma, Alfred, 96, 97, 156
Park, Roswell, 121
Parran, Thomas, 211
Parsons, John E., 21
Paul, Oglesby, 64
Pearl, Raymond, 47, 49, 73
Peck, Gregory, xv, 194, 195
Pendergrass, Eugene, 42, 197, 207, 208
Peters, Vera, 148, 149
Peterson, Reuben, 241
Piazza, Marguerite, 181
Pott, Percivall, 13, 14
Powers, Charles A., 23, 25
Present, Arthur J., 99

Q

Quinn, Luke Cornelius, 212, 213, 219, 223

R

Randal, Judith E., 223, 228, 229, 230
Ranney, Jack L., 174
Rauscher, Frank J., 102, 104, 105, 106, 127, 132, 133, 134, 135, 136, 228, 230, 232
Read, Clifton, 51
Reagan, Ronald W., 194
Reiman, Curt, 204
Reuther, Walter, 200
Reynolds, Edward, 20
Reynolds, Mrs. G. M., 32
Reynolds, James, 22
Rhoads, Cornelius P., 35, 38
Richards, Gordon E., 148
Ringer, Lynn, 176
Robbins, Lewis, 86
Roberts, T. W., 186
Robertson, Cliff, 196
Rockefeller, Laurance, 215, 219, 220
Rockefeller, Margaretta "Happy" (Mrs. Nelson A.), xv, 103
Rockefeller, Nelson A., 103
Rogers, Carrie, 188
Rogers, Edith Nourse, 31
Roosevelt, Eleanor (Mrs. Franklin D.), 211
Roosevelt, Franklin D., 30, 31, 194, 211
Rosenberg, Anna, see Hoffman, Anna Rosenberg
Rosenberg, Saul A., 151
Rosenberg, Steven A., 137
Rosenhaus, Matty, 195
Rous, Peyton, 126
Rubin, I. E., 81
Runyon, Mefford R., 42, 155, 156, 241
Rush, J. E., 24
Rusk, Howard, 212

S

Sarnoff, Dave, 33
Schmidt, Alexander, 232
Schmidt, Benno C., 215, 216, 220
Schmidt, Everett, 176

Schuman, Leonard M., 65
Schweitzer, Robert, 112
Scott, Wendell, 99
Seevers, Maurice H., 65
Seidman, Herbert, 10
Selikoff, Irving, 235
Shapiro, Sam, 100
Shaughnessy, Donald E., 20, 37, 39
Sheahan, Marion W., 64
Shimkin, Michael B., 213
Shultz, George, 220
Silverberg, Edwin, 185
Simpson, Frank, 18
Sjorgen, T. A. U., 19
Snow, John, 13
Soper, George A., 24, 25, 28, 154
Stockard, Charles, 79, 81
Strax, Philip, 100, 101, 102, 103, 104
Sullivan, Ed, 196
Sullivan, Louis W., 188
Sutton, John Bland-, *see* Bland-Sutton, John
Sylvestre, Gene, 175

T

Taylor, Howard C., Jr., 58, 84, 122
Taylor, Howard C., Sr., 16, 18, 19, 58, 241
Terry, Luther K., 64, 65, 66
Thomas, Lewis, 127
Timothy, Francine, 169, 170, 171
Tjalma, R. A., 230
Tocqueville, Alexis de, vii, xiii
Trammell, Niles, 33
Traut, H. F., 81
Tylecote, F. E., 48

U

Ulmer, Thomas, 199, 232
Upton, Arthur, 105, 106

V

Varmus, Harold E., 125
Vidal, Gore, 196

W

Wainwright, J. M., 27
Wallace, DeWitt, 37
Ward, George, 79
Warren, Stafford L., 98
Wasserman, Lew, 215
Wayne, John, xv
Weaver, Harry, 43
Weinberg, Robert A., 128
Welch, Raquel, xv, 196
Welk, Lawrence, 194, 195
White, Jack, 184
Wilcox, Francis (Frank) J., 157, 198, 199, 200, 208, 209
Willig, Armand, 157
Winter, Georg, 17, 18
Wood, David A., 99
Wood, Francis Carter, 20, 212
Woodward, Robert, 227
Woolf, Harry, 235
Worthing, Madelyn, 41
Wydler, John W., 229
Wynder, Ernst L., 49

Y

Yarborough, Ralph W., 214, 215, 219
Young, Joseph, 235

Z

Zubrod, C. Gordon, 143, 145, 146

Index of Subjects

A

Acquired Immune Deficiency Syndrome, *see* AIDS
AFL-CIO unions, 200
AIDS, 136–137
American Association for Cancer Research, 121
American Cancer Society, Inc. (before 1945 *see* American Society for the Control of Cancer)
budget, 5, 39, 124
Cancer-Related Checkup Guidelines, 116–117
Committee on Reorganization (1945), 39
Courage Award, 194–195
dietary recommendations, 141–142
divisions and units, *see* specific names of divisions and units
divisions chartered and incorporated, 39
Foreign Desk, 156
management changes, 43–44, 179
Medical and Scientific Committee, 88
name changed to, 37
NCI, relationship with, 229–230
new Executive Vice-President, 41–44
presidents, 5–6, Appendix C
Public Issues Committee, 234–235
Search committee to replace Executive Director, 42
American Cancer Society, Inc, Board of Directors
business executives/physicians clash, 38–39
chairman, 6, Appendix D
Committee to Advance Worldwide Fight Against Cancer established, 156

divisional representation, 207–209
equal lay and professional representation policy, 6
research grants approval, 124
American Cancer Society, Inc., Crusade Dept., 192–197
Ed Sullivan Show, 196
first campaign (1945), 38
National Kickoff, 194
solicitation of funds *(Reader's Digest)*, 37
This Is Your Life, 196
United Way and ACS, 198–205
Walter Hagen Tournaments, 197
American Cancer Society, Inc., Research Dept.
budget, 124
expenditures through 1986, 7
research grants review process, 123–124
Scientific Advisory Committees, 123–124
American College of Surgeons, 18, 19, 29
American Congress of Physicians and Surgeons, 17, 242–243
American Gynecological Society, 17, 18, 241–244
American Medical Association, 17, 19, 117, 241, 243
American Psychiatric Association, 75
American Society for the Control of Cancer (after 1944 *see* American Cancer Society, Inc.)
Board of Directors, 33–36
cancer research, views of, 121–122
founded (1913), 15
fund raising, 20–21, 33
name changed from, 37
national cancer control, 22–24

organizational background, Appendixes A and B
professional education, 17, 24, 29
professional/lay cooperation, 22
public education, 17–18, 28–30
research policy, 36
survey of state-owned facilities, 26–27
Anderson, M. D., Hospital and Tumor Institute (Houston, TX), 239
Atlas of Exfoliative Cytology, 89

B

Breast cancer, 94–117
Breast Cancer Detection Demonstration Projects (BCDDP), 101, 103, 104–105, 107–111, 114–116, 224–225, 230
breast self-examination (BSE), 96–97
clinical research, 147, 151
controversies, 102–113
General Mills Co. (Minneapolis), BSE project, 205
Halsted radical, 16, 145, 147, 162
HIP (Health Insurance Plan) Study, 100, 102, 104–105, 109
mammography, 98–100, 109
Reach to Recovery, 161–171
risk factors, 95
Vivre Comme Avant, 170–171

C

Campaign Notes, 19
Cancer
death rate, 153–154
Human Values Conferences, 179–182
incidence, 153
Ladies' Home Journal, first lay article on (1913), 19
survival rate, 3
Cancer clinics, 29
Cancer control
definition, 224
progress in, 236–240
Cancer Control Month, *see* National Cancer Control Month (April)
Cancer Facts & Figures, 185
Cancer in minorities, 183–190
Alaskan natives, 190

American Indians, 187, 190
Asians, 190
Black Americans, 184, 185–187, 188–190
Cancer Facts & Figures, 185
Cuban Americans, 187
Hispanics, 190
Mexican Americans, 187
Polynesians, 190
Puerto Ricans, 187
Cancer prevention
controversy, 228
CPS I, 60–63, 65
Pap tests, 91–92
Cancer-Related Checkup Guidelines, *see* American Cancer Society, Inc., Cancer-Related Checkup Guidelines
Cancer research
areas for exploration in (July 1970), 216–219
clinical, 143–152
CanSurmount, *see* Service and rehabilitation programs
Chemoprevention program, 138–141
Chemotherapy, 146–147, 151–152
Cigarette smoking
anticigarette statement (1958), 58–59
behavioral changes in smokers, 73, 75
British Royal College of Physicians Report (1962), 69
and cancer, 47, 67
Committee to review data on smoking and health, 64–65
and coronary heart disease, 67–68
and health, 66, 73
JAMA Hammond-Horn landmark article (1958), 54–55
and life expectancy, 47, 67
and lung cancer, 9–10, 48–50, 53, 56–58, 61, 66, 75
New York Times headline (1954), 53–54
in Scandinavian countries, 48, 69
Surgeon General's Report, 66–67
Cigarettes
advertising, 68, 70
Federal Communications Commission and, 70
Federal Trade Commission and, 68, 70
consumption, 74
filter tips, 54, 75

labeling of, 68–69
sales, 73
tar and nicotine in, 68, 75
Clearinghouse on Smoking and Health,
    see National Clearinghouse on
    Smoking and Health
Clinical Congress of Surgeons of North
    America, 243
Colony-Stimulating Factor (CSF), 138
Colorado Division, 176
Columbia University (New York), 121
Conferences
    ACS National Conference on Breast
        Cancer, 116
    ACS Science Writers' Seminar, 186,
        233
    First National Cytology Conference
        (1948), 85
    Human Values Conferences, 180–182
    International Cancer Congress
        (1933), 155
    International Cancer Symposium,
        (1926), 155
    International Union Against Cancer,
        170
    Meeting the Challenge of Cancer
        Among Black Americans, 187
    World Conference on Smoking and
        Health, 69–70
Consultants, panel of, selected to study
    cancer (March 1970), 215
Cornell University Group (New York),
    82
CPS I, *see* Cancer Prevention Study I
Crusade Department, *see* American
    Cancer Society, Inc., Crusade
    Dept.
CSF, *see* Colony-Stimulating Factor
Cuyahoga Unit, 173
Cytlysin, 138

D

Danger signals (1922), 23
Delaney Amendment, 232–233
Dietary recommendations, *see* American
    Cancer Society, Inc., Dietary
    recommendations

E

Ed Sullivan Show, see American Cancer
    Society, Crusade Dept.

EVAXX, Inc., survey of cancer in black
    Americans, 188–189

F

Federation of Women's Clubs (1932),
    29, 30, 32
Films for black American audiences
    *Five Minutes of Breast Self-Examina-
        tion,* 185
    Time Out for Life, 185
Foreign Desk, *see* American Cancer So-
    ciety, Inc., Foreign Desk
Fund raising, *see* American Cancer Soci-
    ety, Inc., Crusade Dept.

G

Gallup surveys
    ACS's degree of recognition and ac-
        ceptance in, 4
    cost of interviews, 51
    Pap test, 90
    smoking behavior, 73

H

Hagen, Walter, Tournaments, *see* Amer-
    ican Cancer Society, Inc., Cru-
    sade Dept.
Halsted radical, *see* Breast Cancer
Harvard Club meeting (1913), 21, 243
Health Insurance Plan (HIP) study, *see*
    Breast cancer
Hodgkin's disease, 147–151
Human Thymus-Cell Leukemia Virus
    (HTLV), 126, 137

I

I Can Cope, *see* Service and rehabilita-
    tion programs
IAL News, 174
Imperial Cancer Research Fund (En-
    gland), 121
Institute for Cancer Research (Ger-
    many), 121
Interagency Council on Smoking and
    Health, *see* National Interagency
    Council on Smoking and Health
Interferon, 126, 132–136

Interleuken 2 (IL2), 136–137
International Association of Laryngectomees (IAL), *see* Service and rehabilitation programs
International Union Against Cancer,
155, 157, 170–171
Inter-Society Cytology Council, 85

K

Kaposi's sarcoma, 135–136
Kickoff, National, *see* American Cancer
Society, Inc., Crusade Dept.

L

Lasker Awards, 125, 126, 214
Laukoreglin, 138
Lost Chord clubs, 173
Lung cancer, *see* Cigarette smoking

M

Massachusetts Division, 177
M. D. Anderson Hospital and Tumor
Institute (Houston, TX), 239
Memorial Sloan-Kettering Cancer Cen-
ter (New York), 121, 239
Minnesota Division, 178
Minorities, *see* Cancer in minorities
Monoclonal antibodies, 126, 130–132

N

National Cancer Acts (1937, 1971), xvii,
30, 102, 210–222, 227, 239
Conquest of Cancer Bill (1971), 219
President Nixon's State of Union ad-
dress (1971), 220
National Cancer Control Month (April),
194
National Cancer Institute (NCI)
ACS-NCI BCDDP, 102–108, 111–
113, 115
budget, xvii, 211–212, 214
chemoprevention program, 138–141
National cancer weeks, 25
National Clearinghouse on Smoking
and Health, 67
National Institute for Drug Abuse, 75

National Interagency Council on Smok-
ing and Health, 68
National Kickoff, *see* American Cancer
Society, Inc., Crusade Dept.
National Organization for the Study and
Prevention of Tuberculosis, 17
National Research Council
Committee on Growth, 38, 123
NCI, *see* National Cancer Institute
New Voices clubs, 173
New York Skin and Cancer Hospital,
121

O

Oncogenes, 126, 127–130
Ostomy rehabilitation programs, *see* Service and rehabilitation programs

P

Pap tests, 76–93
Pennsylvania State Cancer Commission
survey (1923), 26–27

R

Radiotherapy, 145–147, 151–152
Reach to Recovery, *see* Service and re-
habilitation programs
Rehabilitation programs, *see* Service and
rehabilitation programs
Research Department, *see* American
Cancer Society, Inc., Research
Dept.
Road to Recovery, *see* Service and reha-
bilitation programs
Roper survey, 51
Roswell Park Memorial Institute (Buf-
falo, NY), 121, 239

S

Saccharin, 231–234
Science Writers' Seminar, 186, 233
Service and rehabilitation programs
CanSurmount, 176–177
I Can Cope, 174–176
International Association of Laryn-
gectomees (IAL), 172–174

Ostomy rehabilitation program, 174
programs, 8
Reach to Recovery, 161–171
Road to Recovery, 177–178
Silent Spring, 225
Sloan-Kettering Cancer Center, *see* Memorial Sloan-Kettering Cancer Center
Smoking, *see* Cigarette smoking
Studies
beagle dogs, 71
Bouisson-Tylecotte, 47–48
Cancer Prevention Study (CPS I), 60–63, 65
Hammond-Horn, 50–55, 56–58, 66, 69, 73
high school students, Portland, Oregon, 61
HIP (Health Insurance Plan), 100, 102, 104–105, 109
lung cancer and smoking, 49

T

This Is Your Life, see American Cancer Society, Inc., Crusade Dept.
TNF, *see* Tumor Necrosis Factor
Tobacco industry
political influence of, 59–60
Toxic Substances Control Act (1976), 226
Tumor Necrosis Factor (TNF), 138

U

UICC, *see* International Union Against Cancer
Union Internationale Contre le Cancer (UICC), *see* International Union Against Cancer
United Automobile Workers of America, 200
United Ostomy Association, 174
United States Census Bureau
first cancer statistics, 20
United Way, 198–205

V

Viral research, 125–126, 136–137
Vivre Comme Avant, *see* Breast Cancer
Volunteers, 51–52, 193–197

W

Walter Hagen Tournaments, *see* American Cancer Society, Inc., Crusade Dept.
Wayne County (Detroit) Unit, 200
Women's Field Army, 30–34, 40, 193
World Smoking and Health, 70